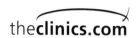
theclinics.com

PRIMARY CARE: CLINICS IN OFFICE PRACTICE

Care of the Older Adult in the Office Setting

GUEST EDITOR
Larry Lawhorne, MD

September 2005 • Volume 32 • Number 3

SAUNDERS

An Imprint of Elsevier, Inc.
PHILADELPHIA   LONDON   TORONTO   MONTREAL   SYDNEY   TOKYO

W.B. SAUNDERS COMPANY
A Division of Elsevier Inc.

1600 John F. Kennedy Boulevard, Suite 1800 • Philadelphia, PA 19103-2899

http://www.theclinics.com

PRIMARY CARE: CLINICS IN OFFICE PRACTICE	**Volume 32, Number 3**
September 2005	**ISSN 0095–4543**
Editor: Karen Sorensen	**ISBN 1-4160-2716-5**

Primary Care: Clinics in Office Practice (ISSN 0095–4543) is published quarterly by W.B. Saunders Company. Corporate and editorial offices: 1600 John F. Kennedy Boulevard, Suite 1800, Philadelphia, PA 19103-2899. Accounting and circulation offices: 6277 Sea Harbor Drive, Orlando, FL 32887–4800. Periodicals postage paid at Orlando, FL 32862, and additional mailing offices. Subscription prices is $135.00 per year (US individuals), $223.00 (US institutions), $163.00 (Canadian individuals), $256.00 (Canadian institutions), $195.00 (foreign individuals), and $256.00 (foreign institutions). Foreign air speed delivery is included in all *Clinics* subscription prices. All prices are subject to change without notice. POST-MASTER: Send address changes to *Primary Care: Clinics in Office Practice*, W.B. Saunders Company. Periodicals Fulfillment. Orlando, FL 32887–4800. **Customer Service: 1-800-654-2452 (US). From outside the United States, call 1-407-345-4000. E-mail: hhspcs@wbsaunders.com.**

Reprints. For copies of 100 or more, of articles in this publication, please contact the Commercial Reprints Department, Elsevier Inc., 360 Park Avenue South, New York, New York 10010-1710. Tel. (212) 633-3813, Fax: (212) 462-1935, email: reprints@elsevier.com

Primary Care: Clinics in Office Practice is covered in *Index Medicus and EMBASE/Excerpta Medica, Current Contents/Clinical Medicine, and ISI/BIOMED.*

Printed in the United States of America.

GUEST EDITOR

LARRY LAWHORNE, MD, Professor, Department of Family Practice, and Director, Geriatric Education Center of Michigan, College of Human Medicine, Michigan State University, East Lansing, Michigan

CONTRIBUTORS

DALE ADLER, MA, MSW, Dementia Care Program Consultant, Fort Myers, Florida

AYHAM ASHKAR, MD, Division of Geriatric Medicine, William Beaumont Hospital, Royal Oak, Michigan

SEKI A. BALOGUN, MD, Assistant Professor of Medicine, Division of General Medicine, Geriatrics, and Palliative Care, Department of Internal Medicine, University of Virginia Health System, Charlottesville, Virginia

HOWARD BRODY, MD, PhD, Professor, Department of Family Practice, Michigan State University, East Lansing, Michigan

MARK ENSBERG, MD, Associate Professor and Clinical Training Coordinator, Geriatric Education Center of Michigan, Michigan State University, Williamston; and Geriatrician, Senior Health Center, Sparrow Hospital, Lansing, Michigan

JONATHAN EVANS, MD, MPH, Associate Professor of Medicine, Division of General Medicine, Geriatrics, and Palliative Care, Department of Internal Medicine, University of Virginia Health System, Charlottesville, Virginia

CYNTHIA GERSTENLAUER, MSN, APRN, BC, Education Specialist, Geriatric Education Center of Michigan, Michigan State University, Williamston; and Nurse Practitioner, Troy Internal Medicine, PC, Troy, Michigan

SARA B. HOLMES, MPH, Coordinator, Education Core, Michigan Alzheimer's Disease Research Center, School of Public Health, Department of Health Behavior & Health Education, University of Michigan, Ann Arbor, Michigan

KATRINA HOPPER, MS, Medical Student (Year 2), College of Human Medicine, Michigan State University, East Lansing, Michigan

KHALED IMAM, MD, CMD, Division of Geriatric Medicine, William Beaumont Hospital, Royal Oak, Michigan

PAUL KATZ, MD, CMD, Professor of Medicine, University of Rochester School of Medicine; Medical Director, Monroe Community Hospital, Rochester, New York

LINDA J. KEILMAN, MSN, APRN, BC, Assistant Professor, Gerontological Nurse Practitioner, College of Nursing; and Faculty Associate, Geriatric Education Center of Michigan, Michigan State University, East Lansing, Michigan

FRANCIS A. KOMARA, DO, Associate Professor, Michigan State University, College of Osteopathic Medicine, East Lansing, Michigan

LARRY LAWHORNE, MD, Professor, Department of Family Practice, and Director, Geriatric Education Center of Michigan, College of Human Medicine, Michigan State University, East Lansing, Michigan

MICHAEL MADDENS, MD, CMD, Chief, Division of Geriatric Medicine, William Beaumont Hospital, Royal Oak; and Clinical Associate Professor of Medicine, Wayne State University School of Medicine, Detroit, Michigan

MARY NOEL, MPH, PhD, RD, Department of Family Practice, College of Human Medicine, Michigan State University, East Lansing, Michigan

KAREN S. OGLE, MD, Professor of Family Practice, Department of Family Practice, College of Human Medicine, Michigan State University, East Lansing, Michigan

KIM PETRONE, MD, Clinical Instructor in Medicine, University of Rochester School of Medicine, Monroe Community Hospital; St. Ann's Community, Rochester, New York

MOHAN REDDY, MD, PhD, Department of Family Practice, College of Human Medicine, Michigan State University, East Lansing, Michigan

CONTENTS

The influx of older patients into the office-based primary care setting is a demographic reality for most practices. A shift from the
disease-driven model of care delivery to one that focuses on function and quality of life should occur if primary care clinicians are to
provide appropriate services to their aging patients. This article
provides an introduction to the concept of incremental functional
assessment and a few practical recommendations about health
maintenance based on the findings of such an assessment. In addition, the emerging public health problem of Alzheimer's disease
and related diseases is explored, as is the pivotal role that office-
based primary care providers can play in addressing the consequences of these devastating diseases.

Information about functional performance is important in caring
for the older adult and complements information about that person's medical status. Knowledge of a person's functional strengths
and weaknesses is necessary to guide decisions about goals of care,
the need for services, and the appropriateness of the living situation. Physicians may underestimate functional disabilities in older
persons, partly because physicians tend to use global rather than
specific measures of function. This article focuses on an incremental
geriatric assessment that is conducted over time by office-based
primary care providers as opposed to the comprehensive geriatric
assessment (CGA) that is conducted in a concentrated manner,
usually by an interdisciplinary team headed by a geriatrician.

time a fall has occurred, significant deficits in physical function already may be present. In addition, a fall is often the consequence of several intrinsic, extrinsic, or situational risk factors suggesting that interventions to reduce the chances of future falls and associated injuries will require multifaceted interventions. This article focuses on ways to identify risk factors before a fall occurs, discusses approaches to implementing interventions that reduce fall risk factors, and examines minimizing the consequences of falls that do occur.

With the increasing number of older adults in the population, the office-based clinician can expect to see more people with urinary incontinence (UI). Continued UI research is warranted that includes older adults and frail elderly women who still reside in the community. Better outcome measures should be developed to assess the effectiveness of interventions for UI. Hopelessness and spiritual distress and their impact on quality of life should be studied in older adults with UI. Improvement in symptoms is demonstrated when education, counseling, support, and encouragement in behavior management and lifestyle interventions are provided. The office-based clinician should ask every older adult about UI and follow with the basic approaches to evaluation and management described in this article.

Hypertension is predictive of a wide variety of subsequent adverse events in elderly patients. Treatment can reduce these adverse outcomes, although the benefits in the very elderly remain somewhat unclear. Target blood pressures in the elderly remain controversial. There appears to be a role for sodium restriction, exercise, and weight loss in lowering blood pressure in some patients. For most patients, low-dose thiazides are likely to be the appropriate first-line pharmacologic therapy unless they exacerbate or precipitate urinary incontinence or gout or complicate concomitant drug therapy. In very elderly patients, the apparent beneficial effects on strokes, major cardiovascular events, and heart failure rates may justify treating despite lack of benefit on overall mortality.

Reconciling best practices in prescribing for older adults who have multiple diagnoses and the potential for polypharmacy and its adverse outcomes can be challenging for the office-based physician.

To successfully prescribe medications for older patients, the physician must be attentive to changes in physiology that may accompany aging and thereby affect the pharmacokinetics and pharmacodynamics of many drugs and the potential drug–drug, drug–disease, and drug–herb interactions. Primary care physicians should also recognize the limited evidence base to support some prescribing recommendations, especially in old or frail old patients, while remaining attentive to those therapies that are effective in this population. Ultimately, the physician must forge partnerships with older patients in an effort to outline goals of care and determine which medications are important in achieving the goals.

This article discusses the recognized risk factors and prevalence of depression and depressive symptoms in the older adult. Emerging evidence supporting the role that subcortical ischemic changes play in the development of late-life depression is presented. Bereavement is addressed briefly, but bipolar disorders are not covered. A systematic process for the recognition and evaluation of depressive symptoms in the office setting is proposed, and a practical approach to treatment and monitoring is described. A guiding principle for treatment and monitoring is that pharmacotherapy without sufficient attention to nondrug interventions is unlikely to be successful.

The purpose of this article is to help physicians who care for nursing facility residents understand their role as care providers in the nursing facility setting. As more care is shifted from the acute care hospital and other sites to nursing facilities, and as the complexity of nursing facility care increases, more is expected of attending physicians. Physicians must structure visits to address patient and family needs and staff concerns; review resident assessment instruments, care plans, and orders for care; and carefully document and code visits to improve the overall care provided to the patient and to assist payers and regulators to have a better understanding of the patient's situation and future plans and expectations.

The elderly comprise most of those in need of palliative and end-of-life care. Nearly 2.5 million people died in the United States in 2002, and three quarters of those deaths occurred in those aged 65 years and over. Five of the six leading causes of death in this age group were chronic illnesses, the conditions most likely to benefit from palliative care. The elderly also represent the most rapidly growing segment of the population, with those aged 65 years and over expected to more than double from 2000 to 2030, when they will constitute 20% of the population. And the number of people aged 85 years and older is expected to more than double by 2030, and more than double again by 2050. Thus the need for palliative care for older adults will continue to rise at a rapid rate.

FORTHCOMING ISSUES

RECENT ISSUES

ELSEVIER
SAUNDERS

Prim Care Clin Office Pract
32 (2005) xi–xiv

PRIMARY CARE:
CLINICS IN
OFFICE PRACTICE

Preface

Care of the Older Adult in the Office Setting

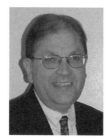

Larry Lawhorne, MD
Guest Editor

The aging of America is upon us. For decades, health care providers gave little attention to the tables and graphs showing the shifting age distribution of the US population while alarmists made dire predictions. But now, with the realization that the first of the baby boom generation will turn 65 years old in just 6 years, the contents of the tables and the trajectories displayed on the graphs give all of us a sense of urgency. The number of Americans aged 65 years and older has grown from 3.1 million in 1900 to almost 36 million today, and is projected to be 71.5 million in 2030. Even more impressive is the number of Americans aged 85 years and over: 4 million today and projected to reach 20 million by 2050.

Many believe that our health care and fiscal systems are not prepared to manage this dramatic growth in the number of older adults. Current analyses suggest that 5% of Medicare beneficiaries consume 50% of Medicare dollars and that many of the high consumers are frail. In addition, there is a shift from acute care needs to chronic care needs, putting many older adults in the waiting rooms of office-based primary care physicians. Already, office visits by older adults make up about 40% of the typical internist's practice, whereas 25% of visits to family physicians are made by people over age 65 years.

Ideal care for the frail elderly may be envisioned as being delivered by a geriatrician and a fine-tuned interdisciplinary team, but this scenario is unlikely to unfold for at least two reasons. First, the cost would be

doi:10.1016/j.pop.2005.06.009   *primarycare.theclinics.com*

prohibitive and second, there would not be enough geriatricians to do the work. Today there are about 7,600 physicians with a Certificate of Added Qualification in Geriatric Medicine in the face of an estimated need for 20,000. Approximately 36,000 geriatricians will be needed by 2030, but the actual number will probably fall far short. This shortfall will place the chronic care of the older adult in the hands of internists, family physicians, nurse practitioners, and physician assistants. As front-line providers in the care of the elderly, these clinicians will need to develop skills in assessment and management of multiple chronic conditions in a single individual and in the recognition, assessment, and management of geriatric syndromes such as falls, urinary incontinence, and dementia. A shift from a disease-driven approach to one that focuses on function and quality of life may be necessary to provide the best care. The office milieu must also allow ample opportunity for the older adult to craft his or her advance care directive.

Although all of this may seem overwhelming, much of what needs to be done comes down to doing simple things consistently and well:

- Ask periodically about key areas of function.
- Ask about falls or fear of falling.
- Ask about urinary incontinence.
- Review the medication list, including prescription drugs, over-the-counter drugs, and herbal preparations; eliminate the ones that no longer have a favorable benefit-to-risk profile.
- Ask about appetite.
- Ask about losses.
- Obtain accurate weights and measure supine and standing blood pressures at every office visit.
- Administer screening and diagnostic tests in an incremental fashion based on what is learned by doing these simple things.

This issue of the *Primary Care: Clinics in Office Practice* is designed to guide the reader through the process of incremental functional assessment suited for the primary care office rather than comprehensive geriatric assessment conducted by a geriatrician and an interdisciplinary team. The first two articles set the stage by providing general comments on the approach to the office care of the older adult and by describing the process of incremental functional assessment. The third article delves into the area of shared decision making because of its importance to much of what follows.

The articles on nutrition and community resources supplement the article on incremental functional assessment. Two common geriatric syndromes—falls and urinary incontinence—are covered next. Injurious falls, especially those that result in hip fractures can be deadly, so reducing fall risk becomes paramount. Urinary incontinence is so common as to be considered trivial or even normal, but its affect on quality of life is far from trivial.

Hypertension is emerging as a major health concern among older adults and may even be a risk factor for late-life depression. Gone are the days when an acceptable systolic blood pressure was equal to 100 plus the age of the patient. The judicious use of the prescription pad is a key factor in providing good geriatric care. Reconciling best practices in pharmacotherapy with the bugbear of polypharmacy is addressed in the ninth article.

The last three articles deal with depression, nursing facility care, and end-of-life care. A most difficult task for the office-based physician is interpreting the meaning of depressive symptoms. Depressive symptoms may indicate that the person is experiencing a major depressive episode but may also be associated with bereavement, loneliness, a medical condition, or the natural disengagement that sometimes occurs near the end of life. What role should the office-based clinician play in the care of his or her patient who enters a nursing facility? If there is a role, how can good nursing facility care be incorporated into an already busy office practice? Finally, clinicians who have the responsibility and privilege of providing care for older adults should become skilled in end-of-life care. As with other aspects of care, good end-of-life care means doing the simple things consistently and well. Communicating with the person who is dying and with family and friends is time-consuming but rewarding. Anticipating and addressing pain and other common end-of-life symptoms are skills that can easily be added to the repertoire of the office-based clinician.

Office-based clinicians are ideally positioned to coordinate the care of older Americans. The skills needed to do it are easily honed, but the time required to do it right is in short supply. In addition, the current Medicare reimbursement system does not appropriately value the care-coordinating activity that can be so important in helping an older adult maintain function and achieve an acceptable quality of life.

As we approach 2011, it can be said that the future is now. Most office-based primary care clinicians will step forward to provide exemplary care for America's aging population. Health care economists and policy makers must also step forward. The executive and legislative branches at state and federal levels must work in a bipartisan way to give Medicare beneficiaries and the health care providers who serve them a health plan that emphasizes function, quality of life, and patient self-determination.

Acknowledgments

Doctors Lawhorne and Ensberg wish to dedicate the article on incremental assessment to Dr. Joseph Papsidero (1929–2000) who was both mentor and friend. We also wish to acknowledge the Bureau of Health

Professions (U. S. Department of Health and Human Services) for supporting the work of the Geriatric Education Center of Michigan.

Larry Lawhorne, MD
Department of Family Practice
Geriatric Education Center of Michigan
College of Human Medicine
Michigan State University
B 215 West Fee Hall
East Lansing, MI 48824, USA

E-mail address: larry.lawhorne@hc.msu.edu

ELSEVIER
SAUNDERS

Prim Care Clin Office Pract
32 (2005) 599–618

PRIMARY CARE:
CLINICS IN
OFFICE PRACTICE

Approaches to the Office Care of the Older Adult and the Specter of Dementia

Larry Lawhorne, MD[a],*, Karen S. Ogle, MD[b]

[a]Department of Family Practice, Geriatric Education Center of Michigan, College of Human Medicine, Michigan State University, B 215 West Fee Hall, East Lansing, MI 48824, USA
[b]Department of Family Practice, College of Human Medicine, Michigan State University, B100 Clinical Center, East Lansing, MI 48824, USA

Office-based primary care clinicians spend a disproportionate amount of time and resources addressing the health needs of their older patients [1,2]. In addition, the cost of providing services to older adults is rising faster than the cost for younger age groups, in large measure because of the consequences of the increasing prevalence of any number of chronic disease states and the expected physiologic changes associated with aging [2].

The entry of the baby boomer generation into the ranks of senior citizens will only increase use of the office-based resources needed to carry out appropriate screening and prevention and to assure the effective recognition, assessment, and management of common medical and neuropsychiatric conditions. In addition, because seniors (like other populations seen by the office-based primary care clinician) are not a homogeneous group, approaches to care based on age alone, on a particular set of diagnoses alone, or even on a specific site of care may not produce desirable health outcomes. Successful approaches to the care of older patients in the office-based setting should focus on assessing and improving function, enhancing quality of life, providing ample opportunity to complete an advance care directive, and honoring the advance care directive after it is in place. Such approaches differ from the disease-driven practice model that has been the hallmark of traditional office-based medicine. Approaches that focus on function, quality of life, and advance planning may require a restructuring of primary care practice and a revision of the methods used to measure provider performance.

This article provides an introduction to the concept of incremental functional assessment and a few practical recommendations about health

* Corresponding author. Geriatric Education Center of Michigan, B 215 West Fee Hall, East Lansing, MI 48824.

E-mail address: larry.lawhorne@hc.msu.edu (L. Lawhorne).

0095-4543/05/$ - see front matter © 2005 Elsevier Inc. All rights reserved.
doi:10.1016/j.pop.2005.06.013
primarycare.theclinics.com

maintenance based on the findings of such an assessment. In addition, the emerging public health problem of Alzheimer's disease and related diseases is explored, as is the pivotal role that office-based primary care providers can play in addressing the consequences of these devastating diseases.

Demographics and office demands

Fig. 1 shows the dramatic shift in the age distribution of the United States population in 1900, 1970, and 2000 and the projected distribution in 2030. As the baby boomer generation (people born between 1946 and 1964) reach the age of 65 years and beyond, what types of health care needs will the office-based clinician encounter? As a preview, consider that about half

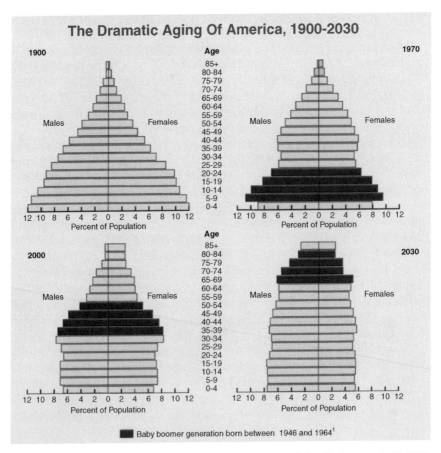

Fig. 1. The shift in the age distribution of the United States population for the years 1900, 1970, and 2000 and the projected distribution for 2030. (Centers for Disease Control and Prevention. Healthy Aging: Preventing Disease and Improving Quality of Life Among Older Americans. Available at: http://www.cdc.gov/nccdphp/aag/aag_aging.htm.)

of all physician visits by baby boomers in 2001 were to primary care physicians, with 16% for preventive care [3]. The top 10 diagnoses for people over age 50 years based on prescriptions written are listed in Box 1 [3]. Hypertension leads the list and, like most of the other diagnoses that appear, has an established, evidence-driven, consensus-based clinical practice guideline addressing recognition, assessment, and management. Most health care organizations and payers encourage adherence to these guidelines, with the expected benefits of reducing disease-specific complications and avoidable hospitalizations [4]. In addition, many of the guidelines have associated sets of quality indicators or other measures that allow comparisons of performance among providers. As the effects of the shift in age distribution begin to be felt in the office setting, however, the fabric of the traditional disease-specific approach to office-based care may unravel for two reasons. First, there are potential pitfalls when disease-specific guidelines are applied to patients with multiple conditions. Second, function and quality of life, especially for people over age 75 years, are often jeopardized by geriatric syndromes such as falls, urinary incontinence, and cognitive impairment rather than by individual disease processes per se.

The potential pitfalls of applying disease-specific guidelines to an individual patient with multiple conditions can be illustrated by a 75-year-old widow who has osteoporosis, hypertension, type 2 diabetes mellitus, degenerative joint disease, evidence of early left ventricular diastolic dysfunction, mild Alzheimer's disease, and depressive symptoms. Implementation of the recommended drug regimen for each one of these conditions individually could mean that she would take over 20 different medications daily, with the concomitant risks of one or more adverse drug

---

Box 1. Top 10 diagnoses for people over age 50 years (by prescription)

1. Hypertension
2. Chronic heart disease
3. Unspecified diabetes mellitus
4. Disorders of lipoprotein metabolism
5. Chronic obstructive pulmonary disease
6. Heart failure
7. Arthrosis
8. Non–insulin-dependent diabetes mellitus
9. Hypertensive heart disease
10. Menopausal and perimenopausal disorders

Data from The "boom" of baby boomers. Available at: http://www.ims-global. com/insight/news_story/0101/news_story_010123.htm. Accessed June 8, 2005.

reactions, one or more potential drug–drug interactions, or one or more drug–nutrient or drug–herbal interactions. Yet, failure to implement guidelines may reflect poorly on a clinician's perceived competence, reimbursement, or both.

The issue of the recognition, assessment, and management of geriatric syndromes is an even more compelling reason to consider restructuring office-based practice in the primary care setting. A geriatric syndrome occurs when an older person with a given set of risk factors is exposed to a new stressor or stressors. A geriatric syndrome, by definition, is multifactorial in etiology, and its successful management requires multifaceted interventions. Continuing the example of the 75-year-old woman previously described, some of the drugs that may have a sound evidence base for management of each of her diagnoses may increase the likelihood of a geriatric syndrome, with its associated decline in functional status and quality of life. For example, the loop diuretic prescribed for heart failure and the angiotensin-converting enzyme inhibitor prescribed for hypertension, heart failure, and diabetes may also contribute to urinary incontinence or a fall. In addition, most health care organizations and payers have not required or encouraged the use of guidelines to address geriatric syndromes and have not implemented quality indicators that measure effective identification or meaningful interventions.

The "Assessing Care of Vulnerable Elderly Adults in the office setting" (ACOVE-2) project describes one approach to restructuring community-based physician practices to facilitate more effective identification, evaluation, and management of three geriatric syndromes: falls, urinary incontinence, and cognitive impairment/dementia [1]. The ACOVE project is an ongoing effort by the University of California at Los Angeles and the RAND corporation that first developed an operational definition of a vulnerable elderly person, then went on to suggest process-of-care quality indicators for community, hospital, and nursing facility settings. For ACOVE purposes, vulnerable elders are defined as individuals aged 65 years and older who are at increased risk of death or functional decline. More information about the ACOVE project can be found at www.acponline.org/sci-policy/acove. ACOVE-2 consists of interventions aimed to improve primary care provided in the community for the three syndromes listed previously by testing four methods of changing medical practice (Box 2). Although findings from this descriptive study are being validated in clinical trials, observations during the ACOVE-2 project suggest that a systematic approach that draws on specific organizational and educational principles can be effective in changing behavior [1]. Fig. 2 illustrates a suggested template for addressing falls or mobility problems. Examples of simple quality indicators for falls or mobility problems that are generated from such a template are listed in Box 3.

How can office-based practices begin to make the transition from the disease-focused approach to a functional and quality-of-life approach?

Box 2. Assessing Care of Vulnerable Elderly Adults in the office setting (ACOVE-2) methods for practice change

1. Efficient collection of clinical data specific to the geriatric syndrome (falls, urinary incontinence, or impaired cognition), including information collected by nonphysicians and automatic orders for simple procedures
2. Medical-record prompts to encourage performance of essential care processes
3. Patient education materials and activation of the patient's (or caregiver's) role in follow-up
4. Support for physician decisions and physician education

Data from Reuben DB, Roth C, Kamberg C, et al. Restructuring primary care practices to manage geriatric syndromes: the ACOVE-2 intervention. J Am Geriatr Soc 2003;51:1787–93.

ACOVE-2 provides some specific guidance with respect to processes of care, but where does the individual clinician start in his or her evaluation of the older patient? Comprehensive geriatric assessment is one potential starting point. During a comprehensive geriatric assessment, the patient undergoes a thorough evaluation of physical function, cognition, mood, gait and balance, medication use, social support, nutrition, vision, and hearing. Comprehensive geriatric assessment, when linked with appropriate referrals and treatment and with adherence to recommendations, is associated with improvements in mortality and quality of life [5,6]. Comprehensive geriatric assessment, however, is not a practical approach for most office-based primary care clinicians because of time constraints. A more feasible approach is incremental functional assessment, which is described in detail in the article by Ensberg and Gerstenlauer found elsewhere in this issue. For purposes of the present article, incremental functional assessment can be described as a process whereby the inability to perform any one of the instrumental activities of daily living (eg, shopping, preparing a meal, arranging transportation, using the telephone, balancing the checkbook, and managing medications) triggers a series of rapid screening tests to determine which domains are contributing to the functional decline: cognitive, physical, psychosocial, environmental, or spiritual. The screening tests and indicated follow-up evaluations can be accomplished incrementally over the span of several office visits, allowing the clinician to determine root causes of the observed decline in instrumental activities of daily living performance, to refine the diagnosis list, and to assign a patient to one of three groups:

- Vigorous and stable (independent with life expectancy at least 5 years)

PATIENT VISIT: FALLS/MOBILITY PROBLEMS

Reason for Visit: ☐ Fall since last visit (or in last year, if new patient) *(MA: Complete Q1-5)*
☐ Fear of falling due to balance/trouble walking only *(MA: Complete Q4-5 only)*

History of Present Illness:

NO

1. Date last fall occurred: _____

2. Circumstances of fall: **YES   NO**
   Loss of consciousness........................ ☐   ☐
   Tripped/stumbled over something........ ☐   ☐
   Lightheadedness/palpitations............. ☐   ☐
   Unable to get up within 5 minutes......... ☐   ☐
   Needed assistance to get up............... ☐   ☐
   ☐

3. Orthostatics: *(Measure after 1-2 min. in specified position)*
   Lying: BP: ____/____ Pulse: ____
   Standing: BP: ____/____ Pulse: ____

4. Uses device for mobility?   **YES**
   Cane...................................... ☐   ☐
   Walker.................................... ☐   ☐
   Wheelchair............................... ☐   ☐
   Other, *specify* : _____ ☐

5. Vision:
   Noticed recent vision change...... ☐   ☐
   Eye exam in past year........................   ☐

   If **NO** eye exam in past year,
   visual acuity today:
   OS: 20/____   OD: 20/____   OU: 20/____

===

6. Psychotropic medications *(specify)*:   **YES   NO**
   Neuroleptics: _____   ☐   ☐
   Benzodiazepines: _____   ☐   ☐
   Antidepressants: _____   ☐   ☐

   7. 2 or more drinks alcohol each day ☐   **YES   NO**
                                                                                           ☐
   8. Other conditions *(e.g., Parkinson's, CVA,*
      cardiac, neuropathy, severe OA), specify:
      _____ ☐   ☐

Examination:

1. <u>Cognition:</u> *3-Item recall:* ☐ **PASS** ☐ **FAIL** If **FAIL** →Cognitive status:

2. <u>Gait:</u> ☐ **NORMAL** ☐ **ABNORMAL**   *If indicated,*
                                                                                                        Timed-

   Up-and-Go: ____sec
   Abnormal if: -Hesitant start   -Heels do not clear toes of other foot
   -Broad-based gait   -Heels do not clear floor
   -Extended arms   -Path deviates

   ┌─────────────────┐
   │ -Stand from chair, │
   │ -Walk 10 feet,   │
   │ -Turn around,   │
   │ -Walk back,   │
   │ -Sit down   │
   └─────────────────┘

3. <u>Balance:</u>   **YES   NO**   *If indicated:*   **YES   NO**
   Side-by-side, stable 10 sec.... ☐   ☐   Can pick up penny off floor........... ☐   ☐
   Semi-tandem, stable 10 sec .. ☐   ☐   Resistance to nudge.................. ☐   ☐
   Full tandem, stable 10 sec..... ☐   ☐

4. <u>Neuromuscular:</u>   **YES NO**   **YES   NO**
   Quad strength: Can rise from chair w/o using arms... ☐   ☐   Rigidity *(e.g., cogwheeling).* ☐   ☐
                                                                                                  Brady kinesia................. ☐   ☐
   If indicated, hip ROM and knee exam: Tremor....................... ☐   ☐

Diagnosis / Treatment Plan / Medical Decision Making:

Lab/Tests: ☐ EKG   **Impression:** ☐ Strength problem   ☐ Severe hip/knee OA
☐ Holter monitoring   ☐ Balance problem   ☐ Other: _____
☐ Other: _____   ☐ Parkinsonism

Treatment:

☐ Patient education handout: ☐ Referral for PT
   ☐ "Falls"   ☐ Assistive device: _____
   ☐ "Home safety checklist"   ☐ Referral for home safety inspection/modifications
   ☐ Strength/balance exercises: ☐ Change in medication(s): _____
      ☐ Upper body   ☐ Lower body   ☐ Referral for eye exam
   ☐ Community resources   ☐ Cardiology consult
☐ Community exercise program   ☐ Neurology consult
☐ Other: _____

Provider's Signature_____

Date of Service_____

See PATIENT CLINICAL SUPPLEMENT: ☐

┌─────────────────────────┐   ┌────────────────────────────┐
│   │   │ Patient Name: │
│   (Medical Group logo here)   │   │ _____ │
│   │   │ Med.   │
│   │   │ Rec.# ───────────────────── │
└─────────────────────────┘   └────────────────────────────┘

Fig. 2. A suggested template for addressing falls or mobility problems. (*Modified from* Reuben DB, Roth C, Kamberg C, et al. Restructuring primary care practices to manage geriatric syndromes: the ACOVE-2 intervention. J Am Geriatr Soc 2003;51:1791.)

Box 3. Possible quality indicators (QI) for falls and mobility problems

QI 1. The prevalence of older adults (>65 years old) who are asked at least annually about the occurrence of a recent fall

QI 2. The prevalence of older adults (>65 years old) who are asked at least annually about the fear of falling due to balance and gait problems

QI 3. The prevalence of documentation of gait, balance, and strength testing for older adults who have had a fall or who fear falling

QI 4. The prevalence of documentation of prescription for strengthening exercises for older adults who have fallen or fear falling and who fail lower extremity strength testing

---

Adapted from Reuben DB, Roth C, Kamberg C, et al. Restructuring primary care practices to manage geriatric syndromes: the ACOVE-2 intervention. J Am Geriatr Soc 2003;51:1791.

- Transitional (physical impairment with life expectancy less than 5 years or moderate dementia with life expectancy 2–10 years)
- Supportive (life expectancy less than 2 years)

After it can be determined which of the three groups is most appropriate for the patient, discussions can be initiated about issues around health maintenance, diagnostic studies, therapeutic interventions, and advance care directives.

Health maintenance

The proper implementation of health maintenance strategies, screening tests, and preventive activities for older adults, especially for those over age 75 or 80 years, can be confusing, with somewhat different recommendations coming from different organizations and associations. By trying to determine the most appropriate group assignment for each patient (vigorous, transitional, or supportive), the clinician can discuss the potential benefits and risks of any of these strategies in an individualized manner.

Several common-sense recommendations have a strong evidence base, especially for those in the vigorous group or the transitional group. Smoking cessation substantially reduces the risk of dying, even for those who quit after age 70 years [7]. Physical activity is associated with decreased risk of death, reductions in the rate of vertebral bone loss, lowered blood pressure, and a reduced risk for coronary artery disease and diabetes [8–17].

Patients in all three categories should be offered annual influenza vaccinations and the pneumococcal vaccine at least once. For patients in the vigorous group or the transitional group whose last pneumococcal vaccine was given 6 or more years ago, repeat vaccination should be offered. With regard to tetanus vaccine, boosters should be offered every 10 years for patients who have had the primary series. For older adults who have not had the primary series, especially for patients in the vigorous and transitional groups, the primary series with a booster every 10 years should be offered.

Table 1 contains some additional health maintenance recommendations developed by an expert panel [18,19]. These general recommendations should be discussed with the patient or caregiver using a shared decision-making approach, supplementing the discussion with the most recent updates from the US Preventive Services Task Force, the American Cancer Society, the American Geriatrics Society, and other relevant agencies, organizations, and associations.

Efforts to convince patients to stop smoking, to exercise, and to keep immunizations up to date are important, as are the activities listed in Table 1. Office-based clinicians should also recognize the importance of doing simple things consistently and well. Taking the blood pressure in supine and standing positions, obtaining an accurate weight at each visit, and periodically asking about falls, fear of falling, and urinary incontinence are essential processes of care in clinics that serve older adults. Finally, implementing processes of care that facilitate the early recognition of cognitive impairment may place the office-based primary care clinician in

Table 1
Selected health maintenance activities

Activity	Vigorous	Transitional	Supportive
Breast examination	Yearly	Yearly	Yearly
Mammography	Every 1–2 y up to age 80 y	Consider every 1–2 y up to age 75 y	No
Pap smear	Consider 1–3 Pap smears if patient has never had one	No	No
Prostate-specific antigen	Discuss pros and cons with patient	Discuss pros and cons with patient	No
Hemoccult testing	Yearly	Consider yearly	No
Colonoscopy	Every 5 y	No	No
Aspirin	If history of myocardial infarction or ≥2 cardiovascular risk factors	If history of myocardial infarction or ≥2 cardiovascular risk factors	No
Medication review	Each visit	Each visit	Each visit

Data from Gerimed Software LLC. Clinical Guidepath tools. Heathrow (FL): Gerimed Software LLC; 2003.

a position to help battle dementia on several fronts: the person with the disease, his or her family, and the community at large.

The specter of dementia

Why is dementia so important? Alzheimer's disease and related disorders have a potentially devastating effect on the functional status of the people who have one of these illnesses. Furthermore, quality of life is adversely affected not only for the person who has the disease but also for family members and friends. Finally, the consequences of Alzheimer's disease can alter the long-standing relationship between the office-based practitioner and the patient who develops the disease. This altered relationship, caused by the cognitive, mood, and behavioral changes that often accompany the illness, affects not only the management of the dementia but also the recognition, assessment, and management of other medical and neuropsychiatric conditions. How common is Alzheimer's disease? How skilled are office-based primary care clinicians in the early recognition and assessment of Alzheimer's disease? How important is early recognition?

Current estimates place the number of Americans with Alzheimer's disease at 4.5 million, more than twice the number in 1980 [20,21]. The numbers are only expected to climb, with projections of a 44% increase by 2025, and perhaps a tripling of today's number by 2050 [20,21]. Not only is prevalence high but the impact of dementia can also be seen in its incidence, which rises rapidly among older adults. Incidence doubles every 5 years starting at age 65 years, with up to 50% of those over age 85 years developing some type of dementia [20,22]. Alzheimer's disease and other dementias account for 40% to 60% of nursing home admissions [20,23]. Direct and indirect costs of caring for people who have dementia are estimated to be at least $100 billion annually [20,24].[1]

In general, the diagnosis of dementia is often not made (or at least not documented) until the patient is well into the course of the disease [25–28]. This observation is partly due to the slow symptom progression of Alzheimer's disease and many other dementias. The symptoms may develop so slowly that they can go unnoticed for several years; if the symptoms are acknowledged, they may seem so slight as to be judged insignificant. In addition, the lack of self-awareness that is part of dementia makes it less likely that patients will report their own problems.

Despite these and other impediments to the timely assessment of cognitive impairment, current knowledge and available evaluation tools can lead to an earlier diagnosis than is now the norm. The office-based

---

[1] For the $100 billion annual cost, this study cites figures based on 1991 data, which were updated in the journal's press release to 1994 figures. Cited in 2001–2002 Alzheimer's Disease Progress Report, July 2003. Publication #NIH 03–5333.

clinician who knows what signs to look for and what follow-up tools are available can act as an effective early warning system. The argument can be made that routine surveillance for early signs of dementia is often key, in that the sooner patients and families receive information, guidance, and appropriate interventions, the better [29].

The effects of appropriate interventions should not be underestimated. Some office-based providers may not be aware of recent changes in treatments for Alzheimer's disease and related disorders or of the effective medications that are available. These medications can be prescribed and managed in a primary care setting.

Given the prevalence and incidence of Alzheimer's disease among aging adults, office-based clinicians should have a low threshold for suspecting the diagnosis. From a practical point of view, some common triggers should raise suspicion even more. These triggers include communication problems, missed appointments, medication management issues, a history of delirium, and more (Box 4). The triggers, which have been divided into five categories, were developed by members of the Primary Care Dementia Network and the Michigan Dementia Coalition. More information about the coalition and its work can be found at www.dementiacoalition.org.

Common barriers to early recognition and diagnosis

Early diagnosis of dementia can make a significant difference in the lives of patients and their families and caregivers, but it is relatively rare that a diagnosis is made early in the course of the disease [25–28]. Most diagnoses are made much later, at a point when the patient is suffering from serious functional and cognitive decline.

The insidious onset of dementia is not the only reason it goes undiagnosed. There also are barriers to diagnosis that relate to patients and their families, physicians and their practices, and the attitudes of society in general. For example, there are individuals who may be so frightened by symptoms of mental decline that they deny them. At the same time, busy office practitioners may perceive the commitment of resources to diagnose and manage dementia to be overwhelming [27]. To the degree that the subject of dementia is considered taboo in our society, it is easy to respond to barriers with silent acquiescence. To a large extent, office-based primary care providers can help overcome these obstacles and the concerns that lie behind them by educating themselves, their colleagues, and the public [30].

One of the biggest concerns is that making the diagnosis of dementia will open Pandora's box, releasing forever a series of problems that will only expand and never be resolved. Given the degenerative course of the disease and its incurable nature, this attitude understandably gives rise to the feeling that the topic is best avoided. Although the frightening diagnosis of dementia might suggest a state of affairs that is beyond control, there are steps that can be taken to improve a difficult situation. A list of barriers to

Box 4. Five main categories of triggers that may suggest dementia

Communication
Consider dementia when an elderly patient
- Misses office appointments
- Calls the office frequently or inappropriately
- Misses paying bills
- Has trouble handling paperwork
- Has difficulty following directions
- Is confused about medication or treatment instructions
- Has difficulty making medical decisions
- Engages in repetitive speech

Accidents
Consider dementia in cases of
- Motor vehicle accidents
- Falls
- Fractures
- Increased frequency of emergency room visits

Medical conditions
Consider dementia when an elderly patient
- Has delirium or a history of delirium
- Has had a stroke
- Has unexplained weight loss

Change in functional status
Consider dementia when an elderly patient
- Has decreased ability to perform instrumental activities of daily living
- Moves to senior housing or assisted living
- Presents signs of self-neglect (eg, hygiene, grooming)
- Becomes less compliant with medication
- Gets lost
- Requires transportation
- Is accompanied to office visits by a family member
- Defers to a family member in answering questions

Cognition changes
Consider dementia when
- An elderly patient or family member reports memory problems
- The patient is unable to list current medications
- The patient is unable to recall recommendations from a prior visit
- The patient is a poor historian

- The patient makes mistakes with medications or the patient's problems do not respond to usual medical management
- The patient experiences late-life depression
- A family member calls before an office visit to inform the physician of concerns the patient may not mention

early recognition and diagnosis of dementia (Box 5) was developed by members of the Michigan Primary Care Dementia Network based on existing literature and using a consensus approach.

Uncertainty about the diagnosis

Because the symptoms of the most common dementia disorders reveal themselves so slowly, over the course of months and years, it can be difficult for physicians to identify dementia in its earliest stage. It may be hard to recognize that a problem even exists, especially when encounters with the patient are isolated and relatively brief, and when no concerns are raised by the patient, family members, or office staff. Even when the suspicion is raised by the patient, family, or office staff or by using a screening tool, recognition of possible cognitive impairment is only a first step in the process. Is the symptom complex that includes a decline in cognition based on of one of the dementia disorders or on some other medical or neuropsychiatric disorder such as delirium or depression? How confident can the office-based clinician be that his or her diagnosis of dementia is correct? If it is dementia, then what is the clinician's confidence level in differentiating Alzheimer's disease from vascular dementia, dementia with Lewy bodies, or one of a number of other causes? Alzheimer's disease is the leading cause of dementia among individuals aged 65 years and older. Alzheimer's disease alone or in combination with vascular dementia

---

Box 5. Barriers to making and documenting a diagnosis of dementia

Uncertainty about the diagnosis
Mistaking symptoms and signs of dementia for normal aging
Lack of appreciation for the benefits of early intervention
Pessimism about disease progression and outcome
Inadequate reimbursement for office care
Patient and family awareness

accounts for 70% of dementia in the over-65-years age group. Given its prevalence, Alzheimer's disease should now be considered a "diagnosis of inclusion" rather than one of exclusion. That is, unless specific, positive findings indicate another form of dementia or a disorder that mimics dementia, it is appropriate for the physician to make a clinical diagnosis of Alzheimer's disease. It should also be noted that Alzheimer's disease may often be present even when other causes of dementia are identified.

The primary care clinician can accurately diagnose Alzheimer's disease and other dementias in the office setting if he or she is alert to common triggers and warning signs of dementia and if easy-to-use cognitive screening tools are employed. Triggers that suggest the possibility of Alzheimer's disease are presented in Box 4, whereas Box 6 lists the warning signs outlined by the Alzheimer's Association. When findings are ambiguous, repeated observations and testing over time usually help to clarify the situation. Given dementia's slow onset, it cannot be overemphasized that this "diagnosis over time" is central to the office-based provider's ability to identify and treat patients in the primary care setting.

Mistaking symptoms and signs of dementia for normal aging

Instances of mild memory loss and cognitive slowing are common as humans grow older: forgetting the location of car keys, occasionally failing to remember a name, or slowing down on some problem-solving tasks. It may be hard at first to distinguish these common losses from the earliest stage of dementia, but when memory deficits or other cognitive deficits start to affect daily function, the distinction becomes clearer [31]. A person might forget the location not only of keys but also of valuable objects; failure to recall names becomes common, and the patient may have trouble remembering the names of close family members; and even simple tasks begin to cause difficulties. As these problems increase, along with declines in organizational ability and reading comprehension, they become more noticeable to family members. In addition, those close to the patient may see signs of behavior changes that include paranoia, withdrawal, or poor hygiene. These symptoms are not signs of normal aging but signs of illness. Erroneous assumptions about such symptoms constituting normal aging should be replaced with increased clinical suspicion of dementia.

Lack of appreciation for the benefits of early intervention

It stands to reason that without a clear benefit, office-based primary care providers would be unlikely to move quickly to establish a diagnosis of dementia. Evidence, however, suggests that addressing dementia early in its course can have a substantial positive impact on the lives of patients and families [29,32–36]. This early intervention applies not only to drug therapies that might slow disease progression but also to the psychosocial

Box 6. Ten warning signs of Alzheimer's disease

1. **Memory loss**. One of the most common early signs of dementia is forgetting recently learned information. Although it is normal to forget appointments, names, or telephone numbers, persons who have dementia forget such things more often and do not remember them later.

2. **Difficulty performing familiar tasks**. People who have dementia often find it hard to complete everyday tasks that are so familiar that we usually do not think about how to do them. A person who has Alzheimer's disease may not know the steps for preparing a meal, using a household appliance, or participating in a lifelong hobby.

3. **Problems with language**. Everyone has trouble finding the right word sometimes, but a person who has Alzheimer's disease often forgets simple words or substitutes unusual words, making his or her speech or writing hard to understand. If a person who has Alzheimer's disease is unable to find his or her toothbrush, for example, the individual may ask for "that thing for my mouth."

4. **Disorientation to time and place**. It is normal to forget the day of the week or where you are going, but people who have Alzheimer's disease can become lost on their own street. They may forget where they are, how they got there, and how to get back home.

5. **Poor or decreased judgment**. No one has perfect judgment all of the time; however, those who have Alzheimer's disease may dress without regard to the weather, wearing several shirts on a warm day or very little clothing in cold weather. Persons who have dementia often show poor judgment about money, giving away large sums to telemarketers or paying for home repairs or products they do not need.

6. **Problems with abstract thinking**. Balancing a checkbook is a task that can be challenging for some, but a person who has Alzheimer's disease may forget what the numbers represent and what needs to be done with them.

7. **Misplacing things**. Although anyone can temporarily misplace a wallet or key, a person who has Alzheimer's disease may put things in unusual places, like an iron in the freezer or a wristwatch in the sugar bowl.

8. **Changes in mood or behavior**. Everyone can become sad or moody from time to time. Someone who has Alzheimer's disease, however, can show rapid mood swings—from calm to tears to anger—for no apparent reason.

9. **Changes in personality**. Personalities ordinarily change somewhat with age, but a person who has Alzheimer's disease can change dramatically, becoming extremely confused, suspicious, fearful, or dependent on a family member.
10. **Loss of initiative**. It is normal to tire of housework, business activities, or social obligations at times. The person who has Alzheimer's disease, however, may become very passive, sitting in front of the television for hours, sleeping more than usual, or not wanting to do usual activities.

Adapted from Alzheimer's Association. Ten warning signs of Alzheimer's disease. Available at: www.alz.org/AboutAD/Warning.asp. Accessed June 12, 2005.

and environmental interventions that may reduce family stress, enhance the patient's sense of control, and promote physical safety.

Pessimism about disease progression and outcome

Without a clear understanding of the benefits that drug treatments and other interventions can bring to patients with dementia and their families, it is easy to view dementia disorders in a pessimistic light. That the disease is incurable and irreversible may seem to be the only relevant factor. Thus, physicians may act (or fail to act) on the unspoken assumption that diagnosis does not matter because "there's nothing to be done." This message may in turn be conveyed to patients and families even when it is not explicitly discussed. A pessimistic outlook leads physicians to not want to talk about dementia and families to not want to ask.

Inadequate reimbursement

The familiar issue of reimbursement that rewards procedures more than thorough doctor–patient communication can be a disincentive to evaluation and management of dementia. Although the incremental assessment process is performed over several office visits, each of which is reimbursable, some of the visits for counseling and the telephone contacts in between will be uncompensated or inadequately compensated given the time and skill involved. The Alzheimer's Association and the American Bar Association Commission on Legal Problems of the Elderly have initiated the Medicare Advocacy Project to gather information and identify problems encountered by beneficiaries and providers [37].

Patient and family awareness

People who begin to experience memory loss and confusion in the initial stage of dementia usually find the experience frightening, but it may be hard for them to share their feelings and worries with family members or health professionals because they believe that naming out loud the thing they fear will make it so. This phenomenon of denial is a defense mechanism that can play a positive role in people's lives, allowing them to digest unpleasant facts at a manageable pace; however, when denial becomes fixed and allows no room for reality to settle in, it stands in the way of a timely diagnosis and of getting the help the patient needs. Just as individuals with early dementia try to hide the symptoms and signs from themselves and others, family members may also practice denial [38]. They also fear for their loved one's future, so they see but refuse to acknowledge the signs of dementia. They might even compensate for the ill person's increasing deficits, offering to share tasks but, in fact, taking them over because the individual is no longer capable.

Benefits of early diagnosis

A diagnosis of dementia is often made well into the course of the disease, when the patient already has serious trouble carrying out daily activities and is showing impaired judgment. The disease has reached a point where family members can no longer ignore or deny it.

What this means in practical terms is that by the time the illness is recognized for what it is, the family may already be in crisis. There may have been an accident, a hospitalization, or a frightening episode in which the person with dementia gets lost. The patient's ability to do basic self-care may be compromised. At the same time, the clinician realizes that it may be too late to initiate medications that might have slowed the patient's decline.

When the diagnosis is made early, at a time when symptoms are present but less severe, it is possible to

- Reduce family stress and burden
- Empower the person with dementia
- Use medications more effectively to improve status or slow progression of the disease
- Help insure the patient's safety
- Identify potentially reversible causes of dementia
- Identify disorders whose symptoms mimic dementia but require a different treatment

Reducing family stress and burden

With good reason, dementia is often called a family disease. As the patient declines, family members must face the emotional stress of witnessing the decline and are faced with new challenges of providing care. Early diagnosis gives individuals with dementia and their families the opportunity to plan for changes before the need becomes urgent. For families especially, the ability to anticipate upcoming changes can reduce the stress of facing an uncertain future and help them cope with those changes when they occur.

Education, care training, and support groups help family members learn ahead of time about the best tools for communicating with their loved one, for providing a safe and comfortable environment, and for controlling difficult behaviors. Evidence suggests that family members who participate in training and support groups are able to care for the patient at home longer [39].

Early diagnosis prepares family members for taking over roles previously performed by the person who has Alzheimer's disease. Early diagnosis also gives family members time to do financial and end-of-life planning in a thoughtful and considered way, often in collaboration with the person who has dementia.

Empowering the person with dementia

When faced with an illness whose course is one of continuing losses— losses of memory, everyday abilities, one's entire sense of self—anything that puts control in the hands of the ill person is welcome. A diagnosis of dementia made early in the disease process does exactly that, affording patients some measure of control by giving them the chance to participate meaningfully in management and planning.

Support groups can help people who have dementia adjust to changes brought on by the illness and empower them to decide for themselves what some of those changes will be [40–42]. Patients can take charge by setting priorities and acting on them and by choosing, to whatever extent circumstances allow, what they will do next. At this early stage, patients can more meaningfully participate in making plans for the future related to finances, caregiving, and end-of-life decisions.

Effects of medication

Information about the effectiveness of the medications that are available to treat the most common forms of dementia is accumulating at a rapid rate. It is now widely accepted that cholinesterase inhibitors and memantine slow the rate of decline in cognitive function in Alzheimer's disease, which may have a positive impact on the lives of patients and their families. Similar benefits have been shown in vascular dementia. The benefits of current medications are real and significant, even when there is no measurable improvement in the patient's symptoms [32–36,43].

The practice of giving a patient a trial of one of these drugs and then watching for improvement is not appropriate. Pharmacotherapy, along with substantive discussion about the drugs, should be offered to every person with mild-to-moderate dementia because it has demonstrated significant value in slowing decline, including delay in nursing home placement. Medications, as part of a comprehensive plan of care, may also be used to alleviate the behavioral or psychologic symptoms of dementia.

Safety issues

It may take a car accident, a fall, or other mishap at home for family members to acknowledge the problems that a loved one who has dementia is experiencing. Even those triggers may not lead to a proper diagnosis if they can easily be explained away as isolated incidents. Early diagnosis of dementia, however, can help minimize the possibility that these accidents will occur. The patient's ability to drive can be carefully assessed, and plans can be made to provide alternative transportation solutions. At the same time, families can begin to modify the home environment for safety.

Identifying potentially reversible causes of dementia

Although signs of dementia most often indicate that Alzheimer's disease or a related neurodegenerative disorder is present, differential diagnosis may reveal other factors that are contributing to or causing the condition. Sometimes these other causes can be treated, thus reversing the observed declines in memory or other cognitive functioning. Differentiating these separate causes sooner means earlier intervention in a potentially reversible illness and greater possibility that the intervention will succeed. Examples of such potentially reversible causes of dementia include metabolic disturbances, vascular disease, thyroid dysfunction, vitamin B_{12} or folate deficiency, infection, and normal-pressure hydrocephalus.

Identifying conditions that mimic dementia

The office-based primary care provider may see patients whose presentation raises suspicion of dementia but who are exhibiting signs of another, treatable disorder. In particular, depression or delirium may be mistaken for dementia in the elderly; however, it is important to be aware that delirium or depression may coexist with dementia.

Summary

The influx of older patients into the office-based primary care setting is a demographic reality for most practices. A shift from the disease-driven model of care delivery to one that focuses on function and quality of life should occur if primary care clinicians are to provide appropriate services to their aging patients, especially as those patients reach a state of vulnerability as defined in the ACOVE studies. Incremental functional assessment may be a first step in making the shift and probably can be implemented in most office-based practices. The specter of dementia, however, is beginning to materialize and affect the approach to addressing the needs of older adults and the expected outcomes of care.

References

[1] Reuben DB, Roth C, Kamberg C, et al. Restructuring primary care practices to manage geriatric syndromes: the ACOVE-2 intervention. J Am Geriatr Soc 2003;51:1787–93.

[2] Wilensky G. Medicare reform—now is the time. N Engl J Med 2001;345:458–62.

[3] The "boom" of baby boomers. Available at: http://www.ims-global.com/insight/news_story/0101/news_story_010123.htm. Accessed June 8, 2005.

[4] Tinetti ME, Bogardus ST, Agostini JV. Potential pitfalls of disease-specific guidelines for patients with multiple conditions. N Engl J Med 2004;351(27):2870–4.

[5] Struck AE, Siv AL, Wieland GD, et al. Comprehensive geriatric assessment: a meta-analysis of controlled trials. Lancet 1993;342:1032–6.

[6] Reuben DB, Frank JC, Hirsch SH, et al. A randomized clinical trial of outpatient comprehensive geriatric assessment coupled with an intervention to increase adherence to recommendations. J Am Geriatr Soc 1999;47:269–76.

[7] US Department of Health and Human Services. The health benefits of smoking cessation: a report of the surgeon general. Rockville (MD): Department of Health and Human Services, Public Health Service, Centers for Disease Control and Prevention, National Center for Chronic Disease Prevention and Healthy Promotion, Office on Smoking and Health; 1990. Publication #DHHS (CDC) 90–8416.

[8] Lindsted KD, Tonstad S, Kuzma JW. Self report of physical activity and patterns of mortality in Seventh-Day Adventist men. J Clin Epidemiol 1991;44:355–64.

[9] Paffenbarger RS, Hyde RT, Wing AL, et al. The association of changes in physical-activity level and other lifestyle characteristics with mortality among men. N Engl J Med 1993;328:538–45.

[10] Blair SN, Kohl HW, Barlow CE, et al. Changes in physical fitness and all cause mortality: a prospective study of healthy and unhealthy men. JAMA 1995;273:1093–8.

[11] Sherman SE, D'Agostino RB, Cobb JL, et al. Does exercise reduce mortality in the elderly? Experience from the Framingham Heart Study. Am Heart J 1994;128:965–72.

[12] Bérard A, Bravo G, Gauthier P. Meta-analysis of the effectiveness of physical activity for the prevention of bone loss in postmenopausal women. Osteporos Int 1997;7:331–7.

[13] Cononie CC, Graves JE, Pollack ML, et al. Effect of exercise training on blood pressure in 70- to 79-yr-old men and women. Med Sci Sports Exerc 1991;23:505–11.

[14] Berlin JA, Colditz GA. A meta-analysis of physical activity in the prevention of coronary hearth disease. Am J Epidermiol 1990;132:612–28.

[15] Eaton CB. Relation of physical activity and cardiovascular fitness to coronary heart disease. Part I: a meta-analysis of the independent relation of physical activity and coronary heart disease. J Am Board Fam Pract 1992;5:31–42.

[16] US Department of Health and Human Services. Physical activity and health: a report of the surgeon general. Atlanta (GA): Department of Health and Human Services, Centers for Disease Control and Prevention, National Center for Chronic Disease Prevention and Healthy Promotion, The President's Council on Physical Fitness and Sports; 1996. Available at: http://www.cdc.gov/nccdphp/sgr/sgr.htm. Accessed April 10, 1999.

[17] Manson JE, Nathan DM, Krolewski AS, et al. A prospective study of exercise and incidence of diabetes among US male physicians. JAMA 1992;268:63–7.

[18] Flaherly JH, Morley JE, Murphy DJ, et al. The development of outpatient clinical Glidepaths. J Am Geriatr Soc 2002;50:1886–901.

[19] Gerimed Software LLC. Clinical Guidepath tools. Heathrow (FL): Gerimed Software LLC; 2003.

[20] Available at: http://www.alz.org/AboutAD/statistics.asp. Accessed June 12, 2005.

[21] Hebert LE, Scherr PA, Bienias FL, et al. Alzheimer disease in the US population: prevalence estimates using the 2000 census. Arch Neurol 2003;60(8):1119–22.

[22] Evans DA, Funkenstein HH, Albert MS, et al. Prevalence of Alzheimer's disease in a community population of older persons: higher than previously reported. JAMA 1989; 262(18):2552–6.

[23] Magaziner J, German P, Zimmerman SI, et al. The prevalence of dementia in a statewide sample of new nursing home admissions aged 65 or older: diagnosis by expert panel. Gerontologist 2000;40(6):663–72.

[24] Ernst RL, Hay JW. The US economic and social costs of Alzheimer's disease revisited. Am J Public Health 1994;84(8):1261–4.

[25] Solomon PR, Pendlebury WW. Recognition of Alzheimer's disease: the 7 minute screen. Fam Med 1998;30(4):265–71.

[26] Cody M, Beck C, Shue VM, et al. Reported practices of primary care physicians in the diagnosis and management of dementia. Aging Ment Health 2002;6(1):72–6.

[27] Carter RE, Rose DA, Palesch YY, et al. Alzheimer's disease in the family practice setting: assessment of a screening tool. Prim Care Companion J Clin Psychiatry 2004;6(6):234–8.

[28] Available at: http://www.americangeriatrics.org/news/alzcons.shtml. Accessed June 12, 2005.

[29] Available at: http://www.alz.org/Care/planning.asp. Accessed June 12, 2005.

[30] Available at: http://www.alz.org/Health/coordinatedcare.asp. Accessed June 12, 2005.

[31] Available at: http://www.alz.org/AboutAD/Myths.asp. Accessed June 12, 2005.

[32] Rogers SL, Doody RS, Mohs RC, et al. Donepezil improves cognition and global function in Alzheimer disease: a 15-week, double-blind, placebo-controlled study. Arch Intern Med 1998;158(9):1021–31.

[33] Wolfson C, Oremus M, Shukla V, et al. Donepezil and rivastigmine in the treatment of Alzheimer's disease: a best-evidence synthesis of the published data on their efficacy and cost-effectiveness. Clin Ther 2002;24(6):862–886; 837.

[34] Tanaka M, Namiki C, Thuy DH, et al. Prediction of psychiatric response to donepezil in patients with mild to moderate Alzheimer's disease. J Neurol Sci 2004;225(1–2):135–41.

[35] Lopez OL, Becher JT, Saxton J, et al. Alteration of a clinically meaningful outcome in the natural history of Alzheimer's disease by cholinesterase inhibition. J Am Geriatr Soc 2005; 53(1):83–7.

[36] Connelly PJ, Prentice NP, Fowler KG. Predicting the outcome of cholinesterase inhibitor treatment in Alzheimer's disease. J Neurosurg Psychiatry 2005;76(3):320–4.

[37] Available at: http://www.alz.org/Health/Insurance.asp. Accessed June 12, 2005.

[38] Teel CS. Rural practitioners' experiences in dementia diagnosis and treatment. Aging Ment Health 2004;8(5):422–9.

[39] Hepburn KW, Tornatore J, Center B, et al. Dementia family caregiver training: affecting beliefs about caregiving and caregiver outcomes. J Am Geriatr Soc 2001;49(4):450–7.

[40] Available at: http://www/alz.org/Research/Funded/2003/03USA_LogsdonIIRG.asp. Accessed June 12, 2005.

[41] Gonyea JG. Alzheimer's disease support groups: an analysis of their structure, format, and perceived benefits. Soc Work Health Care 1989;14(1):61–72.

[42] Gwyther LP. Social issues of the Alzheimer's patient and family. Am J Med 1998;104(4A): 17S–21S; 39S–42S.

[43] Reuben DB, Herr KA, Pacala JT, et al. Geriatrics at your fingertips. 6th edition. New York: American Geriatrics Society; 2004. p. 41–5.

ELSEVIER
SAUNDERS

Prim Care Clin Office Pract
32 (2005) 619–643

PRIMARY CARE:
CLINICS IN
OFFICE PRACTICE

Incremental Geriatric Assessment

Mark Ensberg, MD[a,b,*],
Cynthia Gerstenlauer, MSN, APRN, BC[a,c]

[a]*Geriatric Education Center of Michigan, Michigan State University,
4900 Zimmer Road, Williamston, MI 48895, USA*
[b]*Senior Health Center, Sparrow Hospital, 1210 West Saginaw,
Lansing, MI 48915-1999, USA*
[c]*Troy Internal Medicine, PC, 4600 Investment Drive,
Troy, MI 48098, USA*

Information about functional performance is important in caring for the older adult and complements information about that person's medical status. Knowledge of a person's functional strengths and weaknesses is necessary to guide decisions about goals of care, the need for services, and the appropriateness of the living situation. Physicians may underestimate functional disabilities in older persons [1], partly because physicians tend to use global rather than specific measures of function [2]. To increase physician effectiveness in identifying functional disability, brief but systematic functional assessment of geriatric patients should be integrated into the office visit.

Assessment of a person's ability to function in the home environment requires the examination of several areas of function: cognitive, physical, psychosocial, and spiritual. Strengths and weaknesses in each area are identified. Assessment of the person's social support network must not be neglected, as successful living may be dependent on such support to compensate for identified functional weaknesses. The environment in which the person lives must also be assessed for characteristics that can either facilitate or hinder successful independent living. A model that depicts functioning in the home environment is illustrated in Fig. 1.

Adequate decision-making capacity is necessary to live successfully in the home environment. The presence of acute confusion (delirium) or chronic confusion (dementia) may adversely affect the person's ability to make decisions. In contrast, the ability and willingness to learn new things may have a very positive impact on a person's ability to live successfully at home.

* Corresponding author. 4900 Zimmer Road, Williamstown, MI 48895.
E-mail address: ensberg@pilot.msu.edu (M. Ensberg).

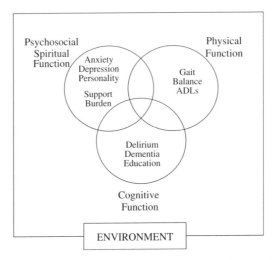

Fig. 1. Successful living at home requires matching the person's functional capabilities with caregiver support and characteristics of the home environment. ADLs, activities of daily living.

The physical skills necessary to live successfully at home include the ability to move through the environment and to provide for one's own personal care. A person may ambulate independently or may require the assistance of a person, cane, walker, or wheelchair. The activities of daily living (ADLs) are tasks related to the provision of personal care: feeding, continence, transferring, toileting, dressing, and bathing. Feeding is the ability to feed oneself after the meal has been prepared. Continence is the ability to control bladder and bowel function. Transferring is the ability to move from bed to chair. Toileting is the ability to use the commode or urinal to empty the bladder, to use the commode to have a bowel movement, and to complete the personal care tasks associated with each activity. Dressing is the ability to entirely clothe and unclothe. Bathing is the ability to bathe in a tub or shower. These activities depend on a person's strength, endurance, and balance. In the later stages of dementia supervision of the ADLs may be required, because the person lacks the cognitive skills to plan and carry out the steps in a given ADL.

Psychologic factors, personality, and spirituality can significantly affect a person's ability to be safe and successful in the home environment. Depression and anxiety are common psychologic factors that can have a negative impact on a person's ability to stay in the home. Personality characteristics may either enhance or interfere with the person's likelihood of remaining safely at home. Spirituality may have a positive influence on a person's satisfaction in his or her environment.

If cognitive, physical, or psychologic impairments interfere with the ability to live successfully in the home environment, the presence or absence of an adequate social support network may be the determining factor in whether a person will remain at home. The caregiver may need to guide appropriate decision-making activities, assist with ambulation, or facilitate provision of personal care. The caregiver may be the person's primary source of psychologic support. The provision of help, however, may present a significant burden for the caregiver. If a caregiver is unable or unwilling to provide this support, then the person may not be able to continue to live at home.

The older adult may live in his or her own home, a relative's home, an assisted living facility, an adult foster care home, or a nursing home. Each of these environments has unique structural characteristics that can affect a person's ability to move through that environment and perform ADLs. In addition, different environments provide access to varying degrees of assistance and supervision with ADLs.

This article describes an incremental geriatric assessment that primary care providers can complete in a stepwise fashion over several office visits. The approach is a three-level assessment process that allows the primary care office-based clinician to administer measures of functional performance in a systematic, cost-efficient manner. Central to the incremental assessment process is the use of assessment tools that are reasonably reliable, valid, and feasible in the primary care environment. Assessment of medical and functional status allows the practitioner to identify groups of older persons who differ in their needs for continuing care (Fig. 2). The approach also provides the practitioner with better information for making medical decisions and with the language necessary to coordinate care. The over-arching goal of care is to assist the older person in maintaining a high quality of life and remaining as independent and safe as possible.

First-level assessment: identify early signs of dysfunction in the home setting

The instrumental activities of daily living (IADLs) [3] are activities instrumental for independent living: using a telephone, meal preparation, housekeeping, managing finances, shopping, and transportation. Difficulty purchasing groceries or preparing meals, for example, may result in poor nutrition unless alternative strategies can be put in place. Poor nutrition may lead to functional problems that accelerate a decline in the performance of IADLs. Therefore, early identification of poor nutritional status or difficulty performing a specific IADL offers the opportunity to identify impairments and to implement interventions designed to assure continued successful independent living.

Step one: recognize nutritional and instrumental activities of daily living triggers

Recognition of an older person's nutritional risk and recognition of potential inability to perform one or more of the IADLs may suggest the

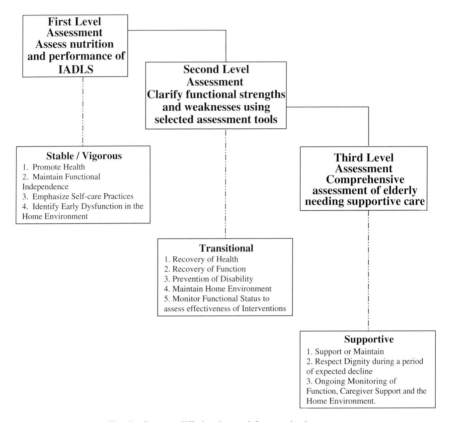

Fig. 2. Groups differing in need for continuing care.

presence of functional impairments that jeopardize the older adult's ability to remain in the home. Nutritional risk or the inability to perform an IADL may be identified by direct observation in the office or by reports from a family member, caregiver, or significant other. This information should always "trigger" a prompt evaluation to identify existing functional impairments in cognitive, physical, psychosocial, or spiritual areas.

With regard to nutritional status, an older adult who looks heavy or overweight may still be poorly nourished. Early symptoms and signs suggesting poor nutrition may not be appreciated because they may be nonspecific or attributed to the patient's established medical problems. The possibility of poor nutrition should be considered if the person has a memory impairment, has had one or more falls, is dependent in one or more ADLs, appears depressed, or is isolated socially.

The person's weight serves as a nutritional screen and should be obtained at every office visit. Even small changes in weight over time may be important. The tendency to assume that weight loss is caused by an unrecognized malignancy or existing or new medical problem should be resisted. Although these possibilities cannot be ignored, weight loss should also trigger questions about the person's dietary pattern, meal preparation, grocery shopping, and social support.

Regarding the person's ability to perform IADLs, showing up for the office visit and interactions related to the visit can be viewed as tests of function. Did the person use the telephone to make the appointment? Did the person drive to the office on his or her own or independently arrange transportation? Did the person come to the scheduled appointment without being reminded? During the office visit, does the person have a good grasp of what the prescribed medications are and how to take them? At the end of the visit, the physician can assess the person's understanding of the diagnoses, instructions, and plans for follow-up. Finally, the person's ability to complete the visit with office staff (eg, deliver the encounter form or billing sheet to the front desk, pay the bill, make future appointments) offers another opportunity to recognize potential impairments that may threaten independent living.

Inquiries about a person's ability to perform the IADLs may identify functional impairments early, before they interfere with a person's ability to live independently. Appendix 2 at the end of the issue includes an IADL form that can be used by the health care professional to facilitate discussion with patients. Self-reports, however, should be interpreted cautiously and should be validated by direct observation or a reliable source in the community, as the older adult may tend to overestimate functional capabilities because of the strong desire to remain at home.

Family members, caregivers, or significant others may express concerns to office staff about how a person is doing. These concerns may be vague or poorly characterized. Discussing specific IADLs provides a language that can help clarify concerns and needs. The older person's current level of function should be compared with prior performance—a few days ago, a few weeks ago, and several months ago. The patient's or caregiver's memory can often be prompted by asking them to recall the person's activities on a recent holiday or special occasion.

Teamwork is essential. Front office staff, medical assistants, and nursing staff should be aware of the triggers mentioned earlier and the importance of suggesting that the physician, nurse practitioner, or physician assistant initiate a prompt evaluation to uncover functional impairments that may threaten the older adult's ability to live safely and successfully at home.

Boxes 1 and 2 summarize the IADL and nutritional triggers that the office-based clinician, patient, family members, caregivers, or office staff should recognize as potential stimuli for additional evaluation. The brief screens that are components of the evaluation process and that should be conducted selectively are discussed later and are included in Appendices 1 and 2 at the end of this issue.

Box 1. Nutritional triggers

IADL related to nutrition
Difficulty with transportation
Impaired mobility and decreased stamina to shop
Decreased stamina to prepare food
History and exam
   "Not eating right"
   Anorexia or poor appetite
   Mouth pain
   Weight loss
   Low body mass index
   Poor dentition
Functional impairment
   Poor memory
   Falls
   ADL dependencies
   Recent losses, depression, social isolation
DETERMINE risk factors [1]

Step two: remember five reasons that contribute to a person's having trouble performing the instrumental activities of daily living

Although a person may develop difficulty performing an IADL for many reasons, most of them fall into one or more of the following five categories: cognitive impairment, physical impairment, psychologic factors, inadequate caregiver or social support, or an unfriendly environment (Fig. 3). For example, a person may not be able to shop for groceries for one or more of the following reasons: (1) insufficient cognitive skills to make a shopping list, find items in the store, or manage money; (2) inadequate physical skills to get from the parking area into the store, push a grocery cart, or carry a sack of groceries; (3) lack of initiative to shop because of depression or anxiety about leaving home; (4) lack of appropriate social support to assist with shopping or lack of finances to purchase food; or (5) unavailability of accessible stores near home (an environmental issue).

Step three: use brief screens to identify potential dimensions of dysfunction

The medical assistant can do a brief assessment of functional status while getting the patient from the waiting room to the examination room by observing whether someone accompanied the person to the office; watching the person get up from the chair and walk to the examining room; weighing the person and comparing current with previous weights; noting if assistance

---

Box 2. Instrumental activity of daily living triggers

Telephone
    Inability to learn use of programmed phone
    Trouble understanding or remembering directions
    Multiple or inappropriate calls
Appointment triggers
    Forgot
    "Too sick to come to appointment"
Transportation triggers
    Episodes of getting lost
    Family comments about reluctance to ride with patient
Medication triggers
    Lack of money to purchase
    Inability to see or comprehend instructions on labels
    Difficulty remembering instructions for medications
    Confusion about number and use of medications
    Inability to remember new drugs
    Inability to take medications correctly, even with reminders
      and pill box
    Fear of side effects or addiction
Difficulty managing finances or business affairs
    "The checkbook was a mess"
    Lack of funds to cover medications
    Impaired vision (eg, inability to read bills, inability to write
      checks)
    Difficulty writing checks
    Fear of spending money even for essentials
    Problems handling money
    Inability to understand bills or statements
    Confusion about due dates and check writing
    Misplacing money, checkbook, valuable papers
Housekeeping
"The house is a mess"

---

is required to disrobe and get onto the examining table; and making observations about the person's general appearance, mood, and demeanor. The patient's medical record should include information about where the person lives (eg, home, apartment, condominium, relative's home, adult foster care, assisted living, nursing home) and should indicate whether the person lives alone or with others. Observations that raise concern on the part of the medical assistant should be communicated to the physician, who should then use selected brief screens of nutrition and function.

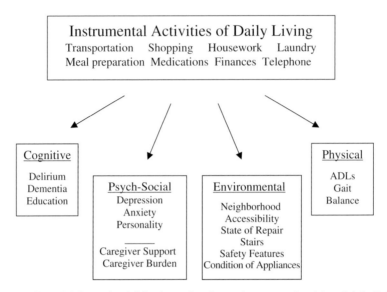

Fig. 3. Differential diagnosis of difficulty performing an instrumental activity of daily living.

Brief screens of nutrition

The one-day food record found in Appendix 1 at the end of this issue is a culturally sensitive way to assess the diet. Ask what the person ate and drank yesterday and if it is a representative account. Ask whether the person eats with anyone else. Note the person's culture, ethnicity, race, and religion. Each of these factors may influence quality or quantity of food and fluids that are consumed. The Determine Your Nutritional Health Checklist (Appendix 1 at the end of this issue) is a useful tool to facilitate discussion with patients and families about nutritional risk.

Brief screens of cognitive function

Evaluation of a person's cognitive function begins with a conversation. The listener must recognize potential barriers affecting communication with the person, including language and culture. Take note of sensory impairments, such as hearing [4] or vision, that may complicate the evaluation. The conversation often begins with a discussion about facts related to that person's medical, nutritional, functional, or social circumstances.

The story that a person tells about his or her current circumstances can provide information about that person's orientation, memory, and insight. The history that is given by a person who has memory impairment may lack specificity or detail or may convey inaccurate time frames. The patient may prefer to spend more time discussing the past than the present, or may look to a family member for help in answering questions. Family members may have a tendency to interrupt and provide answers when the patient has early, perhaps unrecognized, cognitive impairment. Some older adults who have cognitive impairment, especially those who have strong social skills, are adept at hiding their impairment, often using humor as the primary mechanism.

The "Mini-Cog" [5] is a useful brief screen of cognitive function. The Mini-Cog combines an uncued three-item recall and the Clock Drawing Test (Appendix 3a at the end of this issue). The Clock Drawing Test checks constructional skills and executive function [6]. Normal performance for clock drawing is placing all the numbers and the hands in the correct position [7,8]. The Mini-Cog is not affected by level of education or language barriers. The person gets one point for each item recalled after the Clock Drawing Test is administered. A score of zero is a positive screen for dementia, as is a score of one or two with an abnormal Clock Drawing Test. A score of three indicates a negative screen, as does a score of one or two with a normal Clock Drawing Test. The Mini-cog has a sensitivity of 76% and specificity of 89% for the identification of dementia in population-based studies [9].

Brief screens of physical function

An initial brief screen of physical function is an inquiry about falls. Most falls experienced by community-dwelling older persons occur in the home while walking or performing an ADL. Clinicians should ask whether the patient has a fear of falling, as this may be a cause of limited activity. The report of a fall during the night should generate questions about bladder function and toileting. The history of a fall, or a fear of falling, should prompt the check for postural blood pressure changes, evaluation of balance and gait, and a review of medications.

The "Get Up and Go Test" (Appendix 4a at the end of this issue) is another brief screen of physical function [10,11]. Starting in a standard arm chair, the patient is asked to stand from a sitting position, walk across the room about 10 feet, turn, walk back, and sit down. The person should use the customary walking aide. Observe the older person's ability to stand from a sitting position. Note whether the person uses the armrests to push up or requires the assistance of another. Does the person complain of dizziness with standing? A person may ambulate independently or may require the assistance of a person, an assistive device, or both. Is there unsteadiness or sway on arising or when walking? Does the person sway or swerve while turning? Are there signs of gait disturbance? Does the person "plop" back into the chair? Normal time to complete the test is 7 to 10 seconds. Patients who require more than 10 seconds have limited physical mobility and may be at risk for falls. Further evaluation is required if the test is not performed in 20 seconds. See also "Performance-oriented mobility screen" in Appendix 4b at the end of this issue.

The office visit offers the opportunity to evaluate several ADLs, namely transferring, dressing, and (occasionally) toileting. Katz [12] noted that after an acute illness, independence in ADL performance is regained in the following order: feeding, transferring, toileting, dressing, and bathing. When people who have chronic illness get sick, they often lose function in the reverse order. Because the ADLs represent a hierarchy of function, a person observed to have difficulty transferring or toileting must be assumed to have difficulty with dressing and bathing at home, until proven otherwise.

Documentation of a person's ADL performance should include a description of the type and amount of assistance provided. The level of self-performance for each ADL can be measured using the ADL scale in Box 3. Note whether personal assistance or an assistive device is needed. Is mobility impaired because of pain? Observe dexterity, strength, and balance.

Ask about incontinence. Urinary incontinence has economic, psychologic, social, and physical effects on older adults. It is a significant physical impairment that can affect independence and self-esteem.

Brief screens of psychologic function

The history of a loss, including any recent loss of function, should raise concerns about the possibility of depression. Losses may occur in many areas: loss of health, memory, mobility, driver's license, job, income, social standing, spouse, other family member, friend, or pet. Depression can often accompany medical illnesses such as heart attack, stroke, or Parkinson's disease. Depression may follow major surgery or prolonged hospitalization in older patients. Persons who have mild dementia may also experience depression.

Box 3. Definitions for levels of activities of daily living self-performance

Independent
No help or oversight needed

Supervision
Oversight help only
Verbal prompts or cues

Limited assistance
Help limited to physical prompting or guided maneuvering

Extensive assistance
Weight-bearing support
Constant touch or support
Hands-on physical guidance

Total dependency
Full assistance

An effective brief screen for depression is simply to ask one or two questions [13], such as "Do you often feel sad, empty, or blue?" and "Do you have little interest or pleasure in doing things?"

A positive response should prompt further evaluation for depression. Negative responses do not necessarily exclude depression. People will often deny that they are depressed. Therefore, it is important to listen for a history of losses and look for warning signs of depression.

Warning signs of depression can be remembered using the mnemonic SALSA [14]: Sleep disturbance, Anhedonia (inability to experience pleasure), Low Self-esteem, and Appetite decreased. Consider the possibility of depression if there is sleep disturbance. Look for loss of interest or pleasure by asking the person, "What are you looking forward to?" Low self-esteem may present with feelings of guilt, concerns about being a burden to family, and comments about feeling undeserving of blessings experienced in life. Depression should be considered in the presence of poor appetite or weight loss. Other symptoms that should prompt an evaluation for depression include lack of energy, fatigue, decreased libido, chronic pain, or multiple physical complaints.

Brief screens of social support

As stated earlier, IADLs are activities that are instrumental in remaining independent or managing a household. Appendix 2 at the end of this issue includes an IADL form that can be used by the health care professional to facilitate discussion with patients (or families) about potential needs and to review services already in place. Supports may be informal or formal. The informal support network consists of family, friends, and others who do not receive any financial compensation for their work. The size and strength of the informal support network may vary considerably depending on that person's cultural background, among other factors. The formal support network consists of those persons who receive financial compensation for their work, either directly from the patient or patient's family or from insurance coverage or some form of public assistance. All of these supports— informal and formal—may be valuable future contacts if further evaluation or additional support is necessary. The burden experienced by those providing informal support should be assessed periodically.

The brief screens of cognitive, physical, and psychosocial function are summarized in Box 4.

Step four: arrange for medical evaluation and select assessment tools to be used at future office visits

The goal of the first-level assessment is twofold. First, the office-based clinician should identify the older adult who has problems performing one

---

Box 4. Brief screens of cognitive, physical, or psychosocial dysfunction

Nutrition
One-day food record
Determine Your Nutritional Health Checklist

Cognitive function
Conversation
Mini-Cog (three-item recall combined with Clock Drawing Test)

Physical function
History of recent fall
Fear of falling
Get Up and Go Test
Observations regarding transferring, dressing, toileting
Inquiry about urinary incontinence

Psychologic function
History of loss
Responses to two questions about depression
Warning signs; "SALSA"

Social support
IADLs
Identify needs
Inventory services already available in the home

---

or more IADLs or who has nutritional risks or deficits. Second, the clinician should perform the necessary medical work-up and brief functional screens to determine the causes of or contributors to the IADL or nutritional problems so that targeted interventions can be implemented. If the causes or contributors are easily identified and the interventions are straightforward, the patient will not require a second-level assessment and can be assigned to a "vigorous or stable" continuing care group (see Fig. 2). If the patient cannot be assigned to this level of care, the patient should undergo a second-level assessment.

Patients scheduled for a second-level assessment may need additional tests or procedures to evaluate medical or neuropsychiatric reasons for decline, may need to be provided with questionnaires to be completed before the next visit to clarify functional status, or may need to be encouraged to have a family member accompany them to the next visit. The medical practitioner will also need to decide which functional assessment tools will be administered at the follow-up visit.

Second-level assessment: clarify the significance of functional impairments using selected functional assessment tools

The second office visit may include (1) review of observations made at the previous clinic visit; (2) follow-up of an evaluation of medical or neuropsychiatric problems affecting function; (3) administration of more precise measures of cognitive, physical, and psychologic function by a designated member of the office staff; or (4) review of questionnaires provided to the patient or family at the time of the initial visit. In some cases, the observations of a physical therapist, occupational therapist, or visiting nurse will be reviewed. Herewith are listed several examples of the activities that may occur at this office visit. The tools discussed are included in the Appendix at the end of this issue.

Follow-up

Follow-up of medical evaluations should be performed to identify and manage medical or neuropsychiatric problems affecting cognitive, physical, or psychologic function.

Sensory impairments

The Hearing Handicap Inventory for the Elderly [15] can be administered if there are concerns about potential hearing difficulties.

Medication review

All medications (prescribed, over-the-counter, herbals, and vitamins) are brought to the clinic for review. The need for medications that may affect cognition or level of alertness, impair mobility, cause postural hypotension, predispose to falls, or exacerbate anxiety should be re-evaluated. It should be recognized that complex medication regimens may not be feasible in some home environments. For more information, please refer to the article by Petrone and Katz on appropriate medication prescribing elsewhere in this issue.

Evaluation of the pattern of food and fluid consumption

The patterns of food and fluid consumption, which are outlined in Box 5, should be evaluated. For additional information refer to the article on nutrition in the elderly by Noel and Reddy elsewhere in this issue.

Review of the Functional Activities Questionnaire and administration of a Mini-Mental State Examination

The Functional Activities Questionnaire [16] (FAQ) (Appendix 3b at the end of this issue) is a standardized assessment of cognitive activities and is

---

Box 5. Pattern of food and fluid consumption

Usual adult weight
Recent changes in weight
Special diet (type, who prescribed, compliance)
Who prepares food?
Salt added? While cooking? At the table?
Meals and snacks
Fluids during the day
   Alcohol
   Coffee
   Sodas
Eats alone? With others?
Problems affecting intake?
Who does grocery shopping?

---

designed to be filled out by a spouse, family member, or significant other. If concerns about cognition are raised at the time of the initial visit, the FAQ is one of the questionnaires that should be completed between the initial visit and the second visit. Responses to items on the FAQ describe the patient's ability to complete ten complex tasks, including writing checks; assembling business papers; shopping alone; pursuing a hobby or a game of skill; using a stove; preparing a meal; tracking events; discussing a book, magazine, or television show; remembering appointments; and traveling out of the neighborhood. A score of nine or above (out of a total of 30) indicates impairment.

The Folstein Mini-Mental State Examination (MMSE) [17] (Appendix 3c at the end of this issue) is the most commonly used quantitative instrument to screen for cognitive impairment. It has been validated in several languages and cultures. Adjustments for age and education should be made when determining the norms for the MMSE [18]. Sensory deficits can skew results. The MMSE is insensitive to early or mild forms of dementia.

Concordant results on the FAQ and MMSE are helpful in diagnosing or excluding dementia. Discordant results warrant referral for further evaluation. Review of results of the FAQ and MMSE should assist in the diagnosis of dementia using criteria described in the *Diagnostic and Statistical Manual of Mental Disorders, Fourth Edition* (DSM-IV) [19] (Appendix 3d at the end of this issue).

Administration of the Geriatric Depression Scale by a designated staff member

The Geriatric Depression Scale (short form) [20] is a 15-item depression screen that can be administered by a medical assistant or other staff member who has received instruction in its administration (Appendix 5a at the end of this issue). A score of five or more should prompt further evaluation for depression.

Evaluation for depression using criteria described in the Diagnostic and Statistical Manual of Mental Disorders, Fourth Edition

Evaluation for depression should be made using DSM-IV criteria [19]. The diagnosis of depression is made by using specific criteria that can be remembered with the mnemonic SIG E CAPSS [21]: Sadness, Interest, Guilt, Energy, Concentration, Appetite, Psychomotor, Sleep Disturbance, Suicidality. The presence of five (or more) of these criteria during the same 2-week period and representing a change from previous functioning is diagnostic of depression (at least one of the symptoms must be Sadness [depressed mood] or Interest [loss of interest or pleasure]). Using these criteria also provides the clinician with target symptoms that can be used to monitor the treatment of the older adult who has depression. For more on depression see the article by Lawhorne elsewhere in this issue.

Evaluation of anxiety

Anxiety can lead to inability to perform tasks or activities for which the person has sufficient cognitive and physical skill. Anxiety may be related to several factors: medical illness, pain, medication, psychosocial stressors, substance abuse, depression, and dementia. If possible, the best treatment for anxiety is to manage its underlying cause [22–24].

Evaluation for possible substance abuse

Many older adults experience chemical dependency, which affects their ability to function independently. Patients should be routinely asked about alcohol use and counseled about the effects of alcohol, the risks of drinking and driving, and alcohol–drug interactions [25]. Questionnaires such as the CAGE [26] or the Michigan Alcohol Screening Test–Geriatric version (MAST-G) [27] can be used (Appendices 6a,b at the end of this issue).

Evaluation of depression associated with dementia

The diagnosis of depression in a person who has dementia can be challenging, but can be facilitated by using the Cornell Scale for Depression in Dementia (Appendix 5c at the end of this issue). The Cornell is completed by someone who spends sufficient time with the patient to be able to respond to items in five categories: mood-related signs, behavioral disturbances, physical signs, cyclic functions, and ideational disturbances.

An evaluation of decision-making capacity

The determination of decision-making capacity [28] is accomplished by a licensed professional (physician or psychologist). A person is probably capable of making decisions if he or she understands the circumstances, choices, and consequences of each choice, and if the decision is consistent with underlying beliefs and values. The capacity to make decisions is often assessed through conversation with that person. When assessing cognition through conversation, it is important to keep the six C's in mind:

> Communication: are language barriers or hearing difficulties interfering with the clinician's assessment of decision-making capacity?
> Culture: are cultural considerations interfering with the clinician's understanding of the person?
> Circumstances: does the person understand the circumstances?
> Choices: is the person able to state the available choices regarding care?
> Consequences: can the person state the consequences of the choices that are made regarding care?
> Consistency: is the choice consistent with the person's values and previous behavior? Are choices consistent over time? Is the decision voluntary and not coerced?

A person is assumed to be capable of making decisions until proven otherwise. Competency is a legal term; only a judge can determine competency. For more on decision-making see the article by Brody elsewhere in this issue.

Review of progress in physical therapy, occupational therapy, or speech therapy

If a referral was made to any of the therapies or to a home health agency at the initial visit, evaluations and recommendations from these entities should be reviewed and incorporated into the ongoing work-up in the office. Developing a good working relationship with these community-based health care professionals can enhance the assessment of the older adult who is declining; aid in the crafting and implementing of a targeted set of interventions; and later, assist in monitoring the effectiveness of the interventions. The most common limitations to physical functioning of the older adult in the home environment are pain, generalized weakness, and impaired balance, in addition to any functional impairment caused by disease states, such as Parkinson's and stroke. Rehabilitation therapists can be effective in addressing all of these issues.

Fall evaluation

In addition to a previous homecare, physical therapy, or occupational therapy referral, follow-up of a previous visit may include ongoing evaluations and interventions to reduce fall risks [29–31]. Another mnemonic, "Medi-CARE," may be useful: review **Medi-**cations (eg, poly-pharmacy, sedative hypnotics, antipyschotics, alcohol); manage **C**hronic medical conditions that predispose to falls (including poor vision and poor nutrition); treat **A**cute medical problems that increase risk for falling (including dehydration and orthostasis); provide **R**ehabilitative services to increase strength, endurance, and mobility (including an examination of footwear and appropriateness of assistive devices); and correct **E**nviron-mental fall hazards. The article by Komara elsewhere in this issue provides a more detailed discussion of falls.

Evaluation of urinary incontinence

In evaluating urinary incontinence [32], potential causes of recent onset incontinence can be remembered using the mnemonic DIAPPERS: **D**e-lirium, **I**nfection, **A**trophic urethritis/vaginitis, **P**harmaceuticals, **P**sycho-logic (eg, depression, behavioral disorders), **E**xcessive fluid output (eg, high intake, diuretics, caffeine, fluid overload), **R**estricted mobility, and **S**tool Impaction. Evaluation at this visit may include examination of the abdomen, genitalia, and rectum and measurement of postvoid residual volume either by using a bladder scanner or performing postvoid catheteri-zation. Targeted treatment for the causes of recent-onset incontinence often results in resolution; however, long-standing urinary incontinence will require more extensive evaluation and management, which is covered in the article by Keilman elsewhere in this issue.

Follow-up of bowel activity

A follow-up of constipation and discussion of bowel programs should be conducted.

Discussion with a family member, friend, or caregiver

Family members, friends, or caregivers can provide valuable information about an older person's functional status either at the initial visit or a subsequent visit. If the patient is accompanied by someone in the examining room, have the patient introduce that person. Clarify whether that person is the durable power-of-attorney for health care (DPOA-HC), a relative, friend, or caregiver. The conversation should be directed at the patient initially and as much as possible for the entire visit. Always obtain permission from the patient to talk with the companion. Advise both people that if questions cannot be answered by the patient, then the person who accompanies the patient may be questioned later in the visit. Observe the interactions between the patient and the companion. Take time to speak with the patient alone. Family members may be reluctant to express concerns in front of the patient, and vice versa. One strategy may be to ask the companion to step out so that you can spend time with the patient privately, then ask the patient for permission to question the companion. If the older patient is not accompanied by another person, it is necessary to obtain permission to communicate with family. Concerns raised by family members and caregivers should be documented. Communication with others must be conducted in compliance with the Health Insurance Portability and Accountability Act of 1996 (HIPAA) regulations and always with respect for the dignity of the older person.

Home safety

Several home evaluation checklists are available. For patients who have decreased mobility, environmental assessment and modification can promote patient safety and help reduce the risk for falls. The goal of environmental interventions is to identify and eliminate hazardous conditions, and to maximize mobility for the patient. A home safety evaluation by a visiting nurse, physical therapist, or occupational therapist can be valuable.

Based on the results of this second-level assessment, a decision may be made to assign the person to a "transitional" coordinated care group. This care group includes persons who may benefit from interventions directed toward recovery, maintenance of function, and prevention of disability. Persons assigned to this group receive continuing care that is designed to stabilize medical conditions, improve function, and maintain the person in the current home environment. Interventions may include skilled nursing services, rehabilitative services, Meals On Wheels, and personal services provided in the home. Occasionally, short-term institutional placement is needed. Reassessment of the person's medical and functional status is scheduled.

When a person's second-level assessment indicates very low functioning, high dependence on others, or likelihood of decline in functional status or medical condition, then the person undergoes third-level assessment.

Third-level assessment: comprehensive assessment of those needing supportive care

The third-level assessment includes comprehensive measures of function, caregiver support, and the living environment. A profile of the older person's cognitive, physical, and psychologic strengths and weaknesses is made. The home environment is assessed (Appendix 8 at the end of this issue). The functional capabilities of the caregiver may need to be observed, as caregivers may have cognitive, physical, or psychosocial disabilities that interfere with the ability to provide care. An inventory of the informal support network and formal support is made. This third-level assessment may require collaboration with a visiting nurse agency, a geriatric assessment center, services available through the local Area Agencies on Aging, or a private care coordinator.

The home visit may be a necessary part of the third-level assessment and may be provided by the medical practitioner, visiting nurse services, or a private care coordinator. Observation of the older person in the home environment provides the most accurate assessment of that person's functional strengths and weaknesses. The decisions that a person needs to make at home may be assessed by discussing food preparation, medication use, and management of the personal finances. Questions may be prompted by examination of the refrigerator and the medicine cabinet. A person's ability to ambulate, transfer, and perform the ADLs can be observed. Barriers to effective function, such as stairs and clutter, can be identified. Observation of a person's living area, bedroom, and bathroom may identify characteristics of the environment that place a person at risk for falls. Interactions between the older person, family, and caregivers can be observed.

The frail older person's social support network may or may not be able to provide assistance for the cognitive, physical, or psychologic disabilities that interfere with safe living at home. Caregivers may need to provide supervision for safety, guide decision-making, assist with personal care, and provide psychologic support. Provision of this assistance may present a significant burden (Appendices 7a,b at the end of this issue). Conflicting work or family obligations may be a major source of stress and contribute to the burden of care. If a caregiver is unable or unwilling to provide necessary support, then the person may not be able to continue to live safely at home.

The third-level assessment determines whether there is a match among the person's functional strengths and weaknesses, the home environment, and the support network. If the available support and characteristics of the environment compensate for the person's functional disabilities, then continued successful living in the home environment is possible. Efforts should focus on supporting the caregiver and preventing further disability. Arrangements may need to be made for delivered meals or assistance with shopping. The cognitively impaired person may be unable to appreciate the risks of living at home alone, and arrangements for varying levels of supervision may need to be made. For patients who have decreased mobility, environmental modification can promote safety and help reduce the risk for falls. A person who is capable of making decisions may choose to live in a home environment that is less than optimal, and has the right to do so.

Aging and some of the disease processes that are prevalent in older adults are associated with a series of losses that may require significant adaptation and inner strength to overcome. Positive psychologic factors, a strong personality, and spirituality can play an important role in compensating for these losses. Conversely, negative psychologic factors or long-standing personality disorders may hinder the person's ability to live successfully in the home environment. These areas are important to assess as part of a comprehensive assessment. Spirituality provides a means to interpret the meaning and purpose of life. When a person grapples with questions of understanding life choices or circumstances, wonders if there is life after death, and attempts to accept the good and bad experiences of life, then the person is facing personal spiritual issues. Spirituality is also reflected in habits, rituals, traditions, gestures, symbols, and books that help a person manage and interpret life [33].

Based on the results of this third-level assessment, a decision is made to assign the person to the "supportive" care group (see Fig. 2). Persons assigned to the supportive care group will receive a plan of care that includes goals such as (1) stabilizing medical conditions or slowing any deterioration in medical condition; (2) maintaining current level of function or slowing the decline in functioning; (3) maintaining the person at home as long as possible by providing support for caregivers and using community-based resources; (4) modifying the living environment to make it more friendly; (5) changing the living arrangement (placement in a nursing home, adult foster care, or other supervised or assisted living environment); or (6) maintaining personal dignity of the person when death is imminent. A care conference with the patient, the DPOA-HC, family members, and other members of the health care team can be beneficial.

Review goals of care and service needs

As the incremental assessment process moves through the three levels, a clinical decision is made to assign the patient to a coordinated continuing care group. The clinician is aided in making the decision by using tools described to assess the cognitive, physical, and psychosocial dimensions of function. Once this assessment occurs, the functional–medical profile

---

Box 6. Care plan and service needs for the stable or vigorous care group

Advance care directives
Preventive health care [34]
Stabilization of medial conditions
Dietary interventions to maintain or improve nutritional status [35]
Physical conditioning to maintain or increase range of motion, strength, and endurance of the upper and lower extremities
Social inventory and interventions to maintain or improve cognitive stimulation, interpersonal skills, and productive activity
Patient and family education about medical conditions, treatment options, benefits and risks of medications, and likely trajectories of medical conditions and functional consequences
Financial planning
Periodic monitoring of functional status

of each patient is translated into a care plan that specifies self-care and family-care practices and the kinds of health and human services required to achieve the goals of care.

Stable or vigorous

Among individuals assigned to the 'stable or vigorous' care group, the goals of care in Fig. 2 may be accomplished by implementing the service needs listed in Box 6.

Transitional

Examples of the type of services that may be helpful to meet the goals of care listed in Fig. 2 for individual in the supportive care group are listed in Box 7.

Supportive

Examples of the type of services that may be helpful to meet the goals of care listed in Fig. 2 for individuals in the supportive care group are listed in Box 8 [37,38].

Box 7. Potential service needs for the transitional care group

Medical examinations or referrals to identify and treat previously unrecognized remediable conditions and iatrogenic effects of current treatments

Nutrition assessments and interventions

Physical/occupational therapy services aimed at specific objectives, such as improving gait and balance; the ability to bathe or dress; or managing urinary incontinence

Skilled home care for nursing; physical, speech, or occupational therapy; nutritional evaluation; or Social Work Services

Support services, such as delivered meals, grocery shopping, or housekeeping services

Referral for psychologic support
 Support groups for patients or care providers
 Psychiatric medication or psychotherapy
 Other support systems
 Counseling program

Temporary placement in adult foster care or nursing home

Participation in office- or community-based health education/ counseling programs

Monitoring of functional status at defined points in time as indicated by the functional–medical profile of the individual

---

Box 8. Potential service needs for the supportive care group

Neurology, psychiatric, or geropsychiatric referral
Use of community-based long-term care services
   Home health care
   Respite care
   Senior companion program
   Daycare program
   Other adult care services specific to locale
   Homemaker and chore services
   Private caregiving agencies and caregivers
Use of social services to locate the most appropriate living
   environment for persons who have severe functional
   dependencies
Having the patient attend support groups
   Caregivers of aging parents
   Alzheimer's Association
   Specific disease groups
Self-help book referral
   The 36-Hour Day [36]
Caregiver interventions
   Taking care of the caregiver's health
   Encouraging the caregiver to maintain a life outside of
     caregiving
   Counseling
   Having the caregiver share the responsibility with other family
     members
   Addressing caregiver stress or burnout
Ensuring the patient understands the decision-making, legal, and
   financial issues
If possible, maintaining continuity, especially if the patient is
   hospitalized or placed in a nursing home
Frequent monitoring of functional status, social environment,
   and the social support system

Monitoring care

Community-based care is most effective if provided by a health care team that is knowledgeable about that person's baseline functional status. The initial functional assessment serves as a baseline for future comparison. Because the assessment includes measurable parameters, changes in function can be followed over time. If interventions are put into place successfully, then one can look for measurable improvements in function. A decline in function should prompt evaluation for an acute medical illness.

Box 9. Summary of incremental assessment

First-level assessment
Identify early signs of dysfunction in the home setting.
Step one
  Recognize IADL and nutritional triggers.
Step two
  Remember five reasons for IADL impairment.
Step three
  Utilize brief screens of function to identify poor nutrition and
    potential dimensions of dysfunction.
Step four
  Arrange for medical evaluation and select assessment tools to
    be used at a follow-up office visit.

Second-level assessment
Clarify the significance of functional impairments using selected
  functional assessment tools.

Third-level assessment
Make a comprehensive assessment of those needing supportive
  care.

Review goals of care and service needs
Develop and use a list of community resources.

Monitor function and modify care accordingly

Summary

Older adults value (1) independence and the ability to make their own decisions, (2) mobility (the ability to travel outside or simply inside the home), (3) family and friends and the time spent with those persons who are important to them, (4) ethnicity, religion, and spirituality, and (5) home, wherever that might be.

The importance of recognizing each person's individuality cannot be overemphasized [39]. The method of incremental assessment presented in this article and summarized in Box 9 is intended to provide the office-based clinician with sufficient information to make decisions regarding the preventive, therapeutic, rehabilitative, and supportive goals of care. IADL and nutritional triggers are used to identify early signs of dysfunction in the home environment. The strengths and weaknesses of cognitive, physical, psychosocial, and spiritual aspects of function are examined in an incremental manner. Health care providers determine whether there is a match between the person's functional capabilities, the available support network, and the home environment. The approach prompts appropriate use of services needed by older adults who are either at risk for becoming, or already are, chronically ill, disabled, and functionally dependent.

Use of validated assessment tools provides structure for the assessment process, helps assure consistency, and provides a mechanism for periodic re-evaluation. The assessment approaches also foster a common language for the health care team and consist of measurable parameters that can be used to monitor outcomes. The clinician should be flexible and realize that the assessment or the tools may need to be modified depending on the circumstances.

References

[1] Calkins DR, Rubenstein L, Cleary PO, et al. Failure of physicians to recognize functional disability in ambulatory patients. Ann Intern Med 1991;114(6):451–4.
[2] Pinholt EM, Kroenke K, Hanley J, et al. Functional assessment of the elderly. Arch Intern Med 1987;147:484–8.
[3] Lawton MP, Brody EM. Assessment of older people: self-maintaining and instrumental activities of daily living. Gerontologist 1969;9:179–86.
[4] Iezzoni LI, O'Day BL, Killeen M, et al. Communicating about health care: observations from persons who are deaf or hard of hearing. Ann Intern Med 2004;140:356–62.
[5] Borson S, Scanlan J, Brush M, et al. The Mini-Cog: a cognitive "vital signs" measure for dementia screening in multi-lingual elderly. Int J Geriatr Psychiatry 2000;15(11):1021–7.
[6] Tuolcko H, Hadjistavropoulos T, Miller JA, et al. The Clock Test: a sensitive measure to differentiate normal elderly from those with Alzheimer disease. J Am Geriatr Soc 1992;40: 1095–9.
[7] Mendez MF, Ala T, Underwood KL. Development of scoring criteria for the clock drawing task in Alzheimer's disease. J Am Geriatr Soc 1992;40:1095–9.
[8] Esteban-Santillan C, Praditsuwan R, Ueda H, et al. Clock drawing test in very mild Alzheimer's disease. J Am Geriatr Soc 1998;46:1266–9.
[9] Borson S, Scanlan JM, Chen P, et al. The Mini-Cog as a screen for dementia: validation in a population based sample. J Am Geriatr Soc 2003;51:1451–4.
[10] Tinetti ME, Ginter SF. Identifying mobility dysfunctions in elderly patients. Standard neuromuscular examination or direct assessment. JAMA 1988;259:1190–3.
[11] Mathias S, Maual IS, Osaacs B. Balance in elderly patients: the "get-up and go" test. Arch Phys Med Rehabil 1986;67(6):387.
[12] Katz S, et al. Progress in development of the index of ADLs. Gerontologist 1970;10:20.
[13] Whooley MA, Avins AL, Browner MJ. Case-finding instruments for depression. Two questions are as good as many. J Gen Intern Med 1997;12(7):439–45.
[14] Brody DS, Hahn SR, Spitzer RL, et al. Identifying patients with depression in the primary care setting: a more efficient method. Arch Intern Med 1998;158:2469–75.
[15] Ventry IM, Weinstein BE. Identification of elderly people with hearing problems. ASHA 1983;25:37.
[16] Pfeffer RI, Kurosaki TT, Harrah CH, et al. Measurement of functional activities of older adults in the community. J Gerontol 1982;37:323–9.
[17] Folstein MF, Folstein S, McHugh PR. "Mini-mental state." A practical method for grading the cognitive state of patients for the clinician. J Psychiatr Res 1975;12:189–98.
[18] Crum RM, Anthony JC, Bassett SS, et al. Population-based norms for the Mini-Mental State examination by age and educational level. JAMA 1993;18:2386–91.
[19] American Psychiatric Association. Diagnostic and statistical manual of mental disorders (DSM-IV). 4th edition. Washington (DC): The American Psychiatric Association; 1994.

[20] Sheikh JL, Yesavage JA. Geriatric Depression Scale (GDS): recent evidence and development of a shorter version. Clin Gerontol 1986;5:165.

[21] Moses S. Depression screening with SIG E CAPS. FamilyPracticeNotebook.com. Available at: http://www/fpnotebook.com/PSY103.htm. Accessed March 23, 2005.

[22] Banazak DA. Anxiety disorders in elderly patients. J Am Board Fam Pract 1997;10: 280–9.

[23] Cui X, Vaillant GE. Stressful life events and late adulthood adaptation. In: Levkoff SE, Chee YK, Noguchi S, editors. Aging in good health: multidisciplinary perspectives. New York: Springer Publishing Company; 2001. p. 9–27.

[24] Dugue M, Neugroschl J. Anxiety disorders: helping patients regain stability and calm. Geriatrics 2002;57:27–31.

[25] American Geriatrics Society. Clinical guidelines: alcohol use disorders in older adults. Available at: http://www/americangeriatrics.org/products/positionpapers/alcohol.shtml. Accessed July 2, 2005.

[26] Ewing J. Detecting alcoholism: the CAGE questionnaire. JAMA 1989;252:510.

[27] Blow FC, Brower KJ, Schulenberg JE, et al. The Michigan alcoholism screening test: a new elderly specific instrument. Alcohol Clinical Exp Research 1992;16(2):372–7.

[28] Applebaum PS, Grisso T. Assessing patients' capacities to consent to treatment. N Engl J Med 1988;319:1635–8.

[29] Rizzo JA, Baker DI, Mcavay G, et al. The cost-effectiveness of a multifactorial targeted prevention program for falls among community dwelling elderly persons. Med Care 1996; 34(9):954–68.

[30] Tideiksaar E. Falling in old age: prevention and management. 2nd edition. New York: Springer Publishing Company; 1997.

[31] Elderberg HK. How to prevent falls & injuries in patients with impaired mobility. Geriatrics 2001;56(3):41–5, 49.

[32] Penn C, Lekan-Rutledge D, et al. Assessment of urinary incontinence. J Gerontol Nurs 1996; 22(1):8–19.

[33] Sheehan MN. Spirituality in later life. In: Levkoff SE, Chee YK, Noguchi S, editors. Aging in good health. New York: Springer Publishing Company; 2001. p. 41–53.

[34] Takahashi PY, Okhravi HR, Lionel SL, et al. Preventive health care in the elderly population: a guide for practicing physicians. Mayo Clin Proc 2004;79:416–27.

[35] Russell RM, Rasmussen H, Lichtenstein AH. Modified food guide pyramid for people over seventy years of age. J Nutr 1999;129:751–3.

[36] Mace NL, Rabins PV. The 36-hour day: A family guide to caring for persons with Alzheimer's Disease, related dementing illnesses, and memory loss in later life. 3rd edition. Baltimore, MD: The Johns Hopkins University Press; 1999.

[37] O'Brien J. Caring for caregivers. Am Fam Physician 2000;6(12):2584, 2587.

[38] Parks SM, Novielli KD. A practical guide to caring for caregivers. Am Fam Physician 2000; 62:2613–22.

[39] Phelan EA, Anderson LA, LaCroix AZ, et al. Older adults' views of "successful aging"— how do they compare with researchers' definitions? J Am Geriatr Soc 2004;52:211–6.

ELSEVIER
SAUNDERS

Prim Care Clin Office Pract
32 (2005) 645–658

PRIMARY CARE:
CLINICS IN
OFFICE PRACTICE

Shared Decision Making and Determining Decision-Making Capacity

Howard Brody, MD, PhD

Department of Family Practice, B-100 Clinical Center, Michigan State University,
East Lansing, MI 48824, USA

The developments in medical ethics in the United States during the 1960s and 1970s might be characterized as 'the discovery of patient autonomy.' The dominant ethical thinking before that time had focused on the physician's obligation to do good and to avoid doing harm, with "good" and "harm" implicitly being defined according to the physician's own interpretation. The "new" ethical thinking instead focused on the rights of individual patients to make health care choices for themselves, even if they selected courses of action that their physicians viewed as wrongheaded.

Today, the ideal of respect for patient autonomy is captured by the concept of "shared decision making." In a way, this concept represents a melding of the old and new thinking in medical ethics. Like the new ethics, it focuses on the right of the patient to be fully involved in the decision process. Like the old ethics, it focuses on the notion of a shared decision. That is, the physician is expected not to sit passively and allow the patient to choose just any option. The physician is assumed to be an active partner in the process, helping to guide and persuade the patient, so long as the means employed remain on the persuasion side of the line and do not cross over the ethical boundary into the realm of manipulation or coercion.

Shared decision making embodies respect for patient autonomy in a further way. The model allows for various degrees and types of involvement depending on the specific decision to be made and the wishes and values of the patient. Emanuel and Emanuel [1] have helpfully described four models of the physician–patient relationship, ranging from an old, paternalist model in which the physician decides for the patient, to a minimalist model whereby the physician merely provides information to the patient, to more activist models where the physician fulfills the role of

---

E-mail address: brody@msu.edu

counselor, teacher, and friend. In respecting patient autonomy, it is important to understand that demanding that the patient be fully involved in making any and all health care decisions is as much a violation of autonomy as is excluding the patient from decision-making. Some patients want to be more actively involved than other patients, and some patients want to be more actively involved in some types of decisions than in others. Full respect for autonomy entails allowing the patient to delegate various decisions to the physician or others.

Shared decision making as a patient's right implies that the patient is capable of participating in decision making in a meaningful way. Therefore, a focus on shared decision making as a key ethical value in medical practice requires a method by which patients can be assessed for the capacity to choose. It also requires a system whereby decisions can be made on behalf of patients who lack substantial capacity.

The care of older patients becomes especially challenging in relation to these requirements. Various conditions of the elderly can produce dilemmas in assessing their capacity to make medical decisions. Moreover, even when it has been determined that an elderly patient lacks decision-making capacity, what modes of decision making maximally show respect for and promote the dignity of that patient should still be considered. Ultimately, respect for patient autonomy in ethics is not self-justifying; it depends on more fundamental ethical values. One common mode of ethical reasoning grounds the principle of respect for patient autonomy in the more basic value of respect for persons. In the language of the philosopher Kant, we show that we respect persons in part by treating them as ends in themselves and not as means only [2]. Taking away decision-making prerogatives and making decisions for somebody without consultation is a clear example of treating that person as a means only. It would therefore be especially ironic if, in the name of "respect for autonomy," we should end up failing to respect elderly patients by not allowing them to participate in decisions about their own care, simply because they have failed to meet some ideal threshold of decision-making capacity.

Shared decision making, informed consent, and advance care planning

The general idea of shared decision making is that patients who have an acceptable level of capacity should be allowed to make decisions regarding their own health care, to the degree that they wish to be involved in the decision process. They should be able to count on the active support of the physician as adviser and a source of information, and, if they wish and their prior relationship has laid the groundwork, as a trusted counselor and even friend. At any rate, physicians have every right and obligation to try to steer the decision in the direction believed to be in the patient's interests, so long as in the end it is truly the patient's own decision to make.

Two constructs, recognized in medical ethics and by the law, are often the means by which shared decision making occurs: informed consent and advance care planning.

Informed consent means basically that patients have to be given sufficient information to understand their options and the important pros and cons of each option, and then should be asked to consent to a treatment or not, based on how they processes that information in light of their own values and preferences. Informed consent, properly understood, is a communication process that occurs between physician and patient. A signed consent form may be evidence that this process has occurred (and at times is extremely flimsy evidence of this). In no way is the signed piece of paper by itself the ethical equivalent of the actual communication process.

Informed consent implies that a patient is, here and now, capable of comprehending the information and making a reasonable decision based on that information. Many end-of-life decisions, or treatment and placement decisions for elderly patients, have to be made at a time when the patient is no longer capable of that degree of meaningful involvement. An ethical system that values patient autonomy naturally asks whether this means that shared decision making is irrelevant to that entire set of decisions, or whether there is some way to respect patient autonomy even when the patient has lost considerable capacity. The latter option has given rise to the concept first called "advance directives" and now generally renamed "advance care planning."

Advance care planning

Advance care planning makes several assumptions, such as:

At an earlier time, the patient had full decision-making capacity.

At that earlier time, the patient could understand the possibility of various decisions for medical care having to be made at a later time.

The patient understood that at the later time, when the decision had to be made, he or she might come to lack decision-making capacity as a result of illness, dementia, or other processes.

Knowing all this, the patient indicated by some reliable means (eg, verbal conversation, written documents) what decision he or she would wish to be made on his or her behalf at the later decision point, or whom he or she would most trust to make the decision on his or her behalf.

At the present time, the patient has lost decision-making capacity.

At the present time, a decision has to be made that reasonably mirrors the decision the patient had previously anticipated.

The options available at the present time reasonably mirror the options that the patient considered in making his or her wishes known at the earlier time.

Taking all of these factors into consideration, the decision indicated by the patient's prior recorded wishes is respected, or the person the patient had previously designated as the trusted advisor is consulted for decisional input (or some combination of these).

Common decisions made through advance care planning include decisions to employ or forgo various forms of life-sustaining treatment for the terminally ill, including ventilators and feeding tubes, and decisions to admit an acutely ill patient to a nursing home or keep that patient in the nursing home rather than transferring him or her to the hospital.

Debates over autonomy

Much has been done over the past 20 years to facilitate and encourage the use of formal advance directives (living wills and durable powers of attorney for health care), including the passage of a Federal law—the Patient Self-Determination Act. In general, this effort has been disappointing. The number of Americans who have formal advance directives remains in the range of 10% to 20% in most groups, even though many more may have had informal conversations that can be used for advance care planning purposes. This fact has recently led Carl Schneider [3], a law professor, to question the very basis of patient autonomy in modern medical ethics.

In his book, *The Practice of Autonomy*, Schneider [3] compiles impressive evidence to challenge the idea that most patients actually want to participate in health decisions. He succeeds here in normalizing the choice to defer much or all of the decision making to the physician, pointing out that a rational person could have excellent reasons for doing so when burdened by the effects of serious illness. (By contrast, much of the patient–autonomy rhetoric has conveyed the impression that "ethical" people make their own choices and that there is something morally deficient about not wanting full control over these choices at all times).

At the same time, Schneider perhaps overreaches by claiming that there is a serious ethical conflict between the principle of respect for patient autonomy and his empirical conclusions that many patients do not desire autonomy. He views the principle as somehow requiring "mandatory autonomy"; that patients must participate fully in decisions and cannot delegate. This conclusion seems illogical. Any robust principle of autonomy ought to include within it the provision that one may autonomously choose to delegate. Hence, Schneider's helpful empirical survey provides a more nuanced way to apply the principle of respect for autonomy, realizing the wide range of attitudes various patients will have toward shared decision making. Schneider provides no solid reason for abandoning the principle itself.

Schneider also overreaches in a follow-up paper coauthored with Fagerlin [4]. This paper proposes dispensing with one form of advance directive—the living will—again, based on an extensive review of empirical data that undermine many of the assumptions that support advance directives. Fagerlin and Schneider claim to be selectively rebutting the arguments for living wills, while leaving intact the case for the other main form of advance directive, durable power of attorney (ie, appointing a health care advocate or proxy). Actually, their arguments are so sweeping that they undermine living wills and durable power of attorney, and even informed consent itself. They seem to imply that patients cannot possibly become sufficiently informed about a health care treatment choice to know what they would want done to them, unless they have actually experienced the outcome of the choice already; and even if they could know what treatment they want today, they can hardly be sure they will still want the same thing next week. These arguments appear to elevate the undoubted fact that there are practical barriers to fully implementing the concept of shared decision making, coming to the unwarranted conclusion that therefore the concept itself is wrongheaded and useless.

In sum, the bulk of today's bioethics literature favors further efforts to implement shared decision making along with advance care planning as the preferred model, and contrary arguments seem to have less weight.

Determination of capacity

Autonomy cannot be truly respected where it does not exist, and so the accurate determination of capacity to choose becomes a critical feature of any clinical application of shared decision making. The term usually employed in everyday language is "competent." It is helpful to distinguish between patients who are "incompetent" and patients who are "lacking the capacity to choose." The former is properly a legal term. Adults are presumed under the law to be competent until a specific action of the appropriate court finds them otherwise. Also, competence and incompetence are relative terms, and so a court may decide that a person is incompetent for some purposes and competent for others; for instance, competent to make health care decisions but incompetent to make financial decisions.

By contrast, "capacity to choose" remains a clinical concept and requires clinical assessment. If a physician is called to court to testify in a competency hearing, the physician will probably give testimony about the patient's capacity to make various choices, and the court will use that information in deciding competency. Still, it is helpful for clinicians to understand what their job is and to distinguish that from decisions that are properly made by the legal system.

Who can properly determine capacity to choose is also case-specific. In situations such as coma, delirium, or advanced dementia, no specialized expertise is required to conclude that the patient lacks meaningful decision-making capacity. In cases of mild dementia, or coexisting organic brain disease and mental illness, it might be essential that an expert in geropsychiatry examine the patient to determine the precise level and type of capacity. In other cases, detailed neuropsychologic testing might be essential.

The ideal instrument for assessing capacity to choose would focus solely on the process by which one chooses and not the content of one's choice. Value-free criteria would be ideal: one person judging another to have or lack capacity to choose would be objective and would have nothing to do with whether there was agreement with the choice.

This search for objective criteria is a natural reaction to the paternalistic practices of the 1960s and 1970s, in which the mere fact that a patient refused life-prolonging medical care—the mere fact that the patient disagreed with the physician's advice—was taken as evidence that the patient lacked capacity. Unfortunately, this search, at least so far, has proved fruitless. No completely objective set of criteria—no "mini mental status examination" that yields a clear-cut numerical score—has been developed to determine capacity. All capacity assessments include an unavoidable subjective, interpretive element.

The clinical standards suggested by Lo [5] remain an excellent overview of the determination of capacity:

The patient makes and communicates a choice.
The patient appreciates the medical situation and prognosis, the nature of the recommended care, alternative courses of care, and the risks, benefits, and consequences of each alternative.
Decisions are consistent with the patient's values and goals.
Decisions do not result from delusions.
The patient uses reasoning to make a choice.

Lo further suggests that these standards translate into the following assessment questions:

- Does the patient understand the disclosed information?
- Does the patient appreciate the consequences of the choices?
- Does the patient use reasoning to make a choice?

Lo also warns that formal mental status testing and determination of capacity are different functions. At a certain level of cognitive impairment, a patient simply lacks any ability to receive and process health information. But at somewhat higher levels of cognition, a patient might lack specific mental abilities, yet these might not intersect with the mental tasks required to make this particular health decision. At this cognitive level, the patient may possess the needed capacity to choose a treatment plan while at the same time scoring low on tests of cognition. Still, accurate mental status testing is helpful for the clinician who is assessing capacity to choose, because it highlights the patient's specific deficits (such as short-term memory) and points to questions that the assessor needs to ask to be sure that the patient has the requisite capacity.

Making decisions for the patient lacking capacity

The ideal of shared decision making has led to a legal concept that describes how decisions should best be made for the patient who once had decisional capacity but who now lacks it: substituted judgment. Clinicians often understand the legal notion of substituted judgment as something like a "magic wake-up hour."

What the author calls the magic wake-up hour is a thought experiment with these characteristics:

> The patient who currently lacks capacity suddenly "wakes up" for an hour and regains full capacity.
>
> During this hour a full list of all treatment options can be presented to the patient, along with the pros and cons of each, and the patient can comprehend and process all the options.
>
> The patient understands that at the end of the hour, he or she will lapse back into a state of incapacity; and that he or she is making a choice now to determine the fate of his or her incapacitated self (ie, there is an accurate understanding of the true prognosis. If he or she lacks decision-making capacity because of a terminal illness, he or she knows that the illness is terminal).
>
> During the hour of capacity, the patient makes a decision based on accurate knowledge of the facts of his or her case, and based on his enduring, deep values and preferences about how he or she wishes to live his or her life.

This thought experiment comes as close as possible to creating the environment for shared decision making in a patient who now lacks the mental capacity to engage in such decision making.

The notion of substituted judgment therefore suggests a hierarchy of possible decisions a clinician might make on behalf of the incapacitated individual:

> Clinicians allow the decision to be made by the person designated formally by the patient through a durable power of attorney.
>
> Clinicians choose according to directions written down by the patient in the form of a document (eg, living will).
>
> Clinicians allow the decision to be made by a "natural" proxy, such as the patient's legal next of kin, based on previous, informal conversations in which the patient conveyed his wishes.
>
> Clinicians allow the decision to be made by a "natural" proxy, such as the patient's legal next of kin, based on their general knowledge of the patient as a person, but without having had any focused conversations about health care choices.
>
> Clinicians choose based on their subjective judgment about the patient's future quality of life, in the absence of any proxy or previously recorded wishes.

Proceeding downward through the hierarchy, two variables decrease in value: the level of confidence that the choice reflects the patient's "true" wishes, and the extent to which the clinician can invoke the principle of respect for autonomy in justifying their choice. In levels one and two of the hierarchy, it would seem that the patient's autonomous wishes are being expressed on his behalf. By the time level five is reached, the notion of autonomy is largely irrelevant. The clinician is doing the best he or she can for the patient, but the choice has virtually nothing to do with the patient's autonomy or prior wishes, which remain unknown in such cases.

Mr. Smith doesn't live here anymore

Some of the most emotionally difficult cases involving the elderly unfold roughly like the scenario illustrated as follows.

All through his life, Mr. Smith adamantly prided himself most for his mental acumen; his ability to think and communicate. He told his family and recorded in a living will that he would rather be dead than a demented person in a nursing home, unable to recognize his friends and family, unaware of the current events of the day.

He then suffered a series of small strokes and developed a dementia of the Alzheimer type. At no time did he have a specific health crisis in which a decision had to be made about a ventilator or other life support. However, he gradually developed more and more physical and mental limitations. It became impossible for him to be cared for at home and he eventually required admission to an extended care facility.

He is now in precisely the state he once said was worse than death. But he presently appears to be content with his current experiences. He watches people walk by, looks out the window at the trees and birds, and smiles at all who greet him. He shows no sign of pain or distress. He blissfully seems to have no recollection of his former self who railed against the existence he now has.

The staff members who care for Mr. Smith feel it would be an outrage to deny him care if, for instance, he developed a pneumonia that could be easily reversed by antibiotics. A nephew who is now his legal guardian understands the staff's point of view and primarily sympathizes with them. But the nephew also feels some duty to carry out Mr. Smith's clearly expressed, prior wishes [6].

How could it be explained to the staff and the nephew what the ideal of shared decision making requires of them in Mr. Smith's case?

One way to approach this problem is to imagine that somehow the same human body has come to be occupied in succession by two different persons, who might be called Smith One and Smith Two. Smith One possessed decision-making capacity and made known his wishes through the living will and other means. Smith Two lacks decision-making capacity and unlike Smith One, appears to be content to survive in a state of radically diminished mental function. Smith Two, lacking decisional capacity and being physically frail, is an especially vulnerable individual and must depend on his clinicians to protect his interests, whatever those interests may be.

This approach to the problem sets up two opposite resolutions.

First resolution

Respect for autonomy requires that the wishes of Smith One are honored. He had full mental capacity when he registered those wishes. Above all else, Smith One wished not to be condemned to live out an existence like the one now experienced by Smith Two. If Smith Two is kept alive through medical interventions, Smith One is condemned to the fate he most feared.

Smith One has in a sense ceased to exist; but in another sense, he lives on in Smith Two's body. Smith Two's body is the only living and visible memory of Smith One that can be seen by his surviving friends and family. When Smith One expressed his wishes for his future, he was not merely saying what kinds of experiences he wished to have, he was also making a statement about how he wanted to be remembered by his survivors. The only way to honor his wishes in this matter is to regard Smith Two's body as still belonging to Smith One and therefore governed by Smith One's recorded choices.

Second resolution

Smith One, as a person, no longer exists. Therefore there is no longer any effective way to honor Smith One's autonomy. But Smith One's body is currently inhabited by Smith Two. Smith Two seems to be enjoying his somewhat limited life and there is no justification for terminating his existence. To allow Smith Two to die prematurely, in accord with wishes expressed by Smith One, would be a violation of duties owed to Smith Two.

Moreover, if the clinician agrees to allow Smith Two to die based on Smith One's previously expressed wishes, he is engaging in an especially invidious form of discrimination against persons who have disabilities. Smith Two has certain disabilities, and Smith One didn't want such a person to live specifically because Smith One viewed the life of such a person as less worthy or less deserving than the life of a person who has full mental capacity (ie, the life of a nondisabled person). But this is a totally inappropriate moral framework from which to make life and death decisions about Smith Two [7].

Just to complicate matters, a third resolution may be suggested.

Third resolution

The first and second resolutions actually destroy Smith's basic dignity as a person, because they rely on an unacceptable premise—the notion that

Smith can be artificially divided into two different people. The idea that Smith One no longer exists and that Smith Two has taken his place essentially depends on a particular model of personhood that might be termed "person-as-mind." According to this view, being a person requires certain mental capabilities, and one loses personhood when one loses those capabilities. But reducing the full human person to only mental processes is a truncated and inadequate way of viewing the person.

By contrast, Smith's nephew seems to have at least a glimmer of a better model of personhood, which might be termed "person-as-nested-in-relationships." The nephew is torn because he wishes to honor who his uncle used to be, but he worries about the vulnerability of his uncle as he is now. What makes these the same person is that they are both his uncle. Smith remains in the same relationships with his family and friends despite his developing mental incapacity. The question, "How can I most compassionately take care of my uncle?" may be a much better (if still ambiguous) ethical guide to the nephew than artificial resolutions concocted at the expense of Smith's basic human dignity.

Respecting the dignity of incapacitated elderly

Deep metaphysical issues about what it means to be a human person are clearly beyond the scope of this article. But there are some well-articulated ethical reasons for not discounting Smith's present life experience in making medical decisions, and therefore not giving automatic or complete priority to Smith's advance directive. How best to do so, without violating Smith's right as a person who has capacity to take control of his future destiny, could become problematic. But what it means to take Smith's present life experiences seriously while still acknowledging his present incapacity needs to be explored.

Dresser and Whitehouse [8] offer one of the most thorough discussions of using the life experiences of the incapacitated elderly to guide at least some medical treatment decisions. They focus especially on the subjective determination of the patient's present, experiential values. The ethical value of assent can be added to that.

The discussion of what the present Mr. Smith (Smith Two) appears to enjoy doing illustrates the notion of the subjective determination of Smith's experiential values. A person who carefully and sympathetically watches Mr. Smith in his present environment can make several well-grounded judgments about what Mr. Smith currently values in his life. If two caregivers disagreed about something (eg, whether Mr. Smith prefers split pea soup to clam chowder or vice versa), they might develop ways to get evidence to settle this disagreement. Many decisions about Mr. Smith's day-to-day care can be resolved by an appeal to his present structure of lived values.

The point urged by Dresser and Whitehouse is that we should not allow our fixation with decisional capacity to discount these determinations of present values simply because Mr. Smith now lacks decisional capacity. It is easy to decide that Mr. Smith's living will, in which he formally declared that he would not want to be kept alive in this state, conclusively "trumps" any nonsense about which soup the demented Mr. Smith now seems to favor. But this attitude could lead to what amounts to: "I will respect your dignity as a human being only so long as you possess full decisional capacity, but will stop respecting your dignity as soon as you lose that capacity." The goal in ethical decision making should be a full measure of respect for the dignity of all patients, including those who have ceased to have capacity. And that in turn requires close consideration of the life they are experiencing today and what medical treatment decisions might best cohere with the values that are discerned.

It is important to note that such attention to lived experience will not necessarily translate into an ethical stance of always prolonging life. In the difficult case of Mr. Smith, there is a direct clash between two contrary ethical reasons: the advance directive, favoring no life-prolonging therapy, and Mr. Smith's current experiential values, favoring at least some efforts to extend his life. In other cases, a careful assessment of the patient's lived experience may dictate that a life-prolonging therapy should not be administered. A common example from an older time (it is hoped) is the patient who continues to pull out gastrostomy tubes, and so ends up with a gastrostomy tube in place and his or her hands tied so that he or she cannot pull it out. The need to tie down the patient's hands to keep the tube in place should trigger a sober assessment of what quality of life the tube is going to produce that could possibly be worth the extreme deterioration in quality of life that the tied hands will produce. In still other cases, the best assessment of the patient's current lived experience is his or her indifference to the length of time he or she goes on living. In such a case, an advance directive would then clearly outweigh any other ethical considerations.

The importance of patient assent is another way to preserve the dignity of the older patient. A roughly analogous concept applies to children. Infants cannot give either consent or assent. Clinicians do what they believe needs to be done, whether the child cries or not. An adolescent aged 15 or 16 years probably has the mental capacity to give as valid an informed consent as an adult (even if not legally empowered to do so). In between infancy and adolescence, children may not be given the right to consent to medical care, but their right to assent is respected whenever possible. The 8-year-old who has leukemia is not allowed to veto her lumbar puncture, but neither is she simply dragged screaming into the room and held down for the procedure. Every attempt would be made to persuade her to accept the painful procedure and to comply voluntarily.

Although it may seem undignified to compare elderly patients to children, the concept of assent can still play a role in the respectful treatment of these patients. A general rule of trying to seek patient assent, even where a true informed consent cannot be obtained, seems to be a valid way to express respect. The problem today may be less with individual actions that violate patient assent, and more with institutional patterns of activity that discount assent and treat patients as objects to be moved from one place to another at the will of the staff. Over time, in such an institutional setting, the staff and the patients themselves can gradually lose sight of the fact that patients are human beings deserving of dignified treatment. The same might occur in a home care situation if, for example, the administrative requirements of the home health agency (such as fear of liability if the caregivers are unable to ensure a safe home environment) are allowed to overwhelm a realistic assessment of the patient's preferences and practical options (which might include accepting the risk of staying in a somewhat unsafe home rather than being admitted to an institution).

Summary: the current culture of biomedicine and aging

The dominant stream in current bioethical thinking focuses on shared decision making, which in turn seems to stress the concept of individual choice. This collection of ideas implies that elderly patients and their families can engage in meaningful choices concerning end-of-life care. A sobering but helpful commentary calls the mythology of individual choice into question.

Kaufman and colleagues [9] remind us that we live in a society and a culture. We might imagine that we can make choices, but the social and cultural environment sends us powerful messages about what is expected of us; what is open to personal choice and what is not. Certain options for the care of elderly patients may be matters of choice according to bioethical theory, yet be effectively moved off the table in a social and cultural setting that simply takes for granted that people involved in the care of an elderly patient will act in some ways and not in others.

The cultural environment on which Kaufman and colleagues want to focus the attention of the geriatrics community is what they call the "biomedicalization of aging." This concept was formally introduced by Estes and Binney [10] in 1989. It was also implicit in the controversial book, *Setting Limits*, by bioethicist and philosopher Daniel Callahan [11] in 1987. Callahan's book initially stirred controversy because of his proposal that after a certain age, elderly patients should no longer have the right to receive life-extending medical care and should instead be entitled only to care that promotes comfort and quality of life. But his deeper message was a warning that Western society had profoundly shifted its ground in how it addressed the idea of aging and mortality. No longer comfortable with an explicitly religious framework in which aging and death are accepted as part of the Divine plan, our society (Callahan asserted) has sought to assuage or eliminate our fears of growing old and dying by turning those life processes into technologic problems. We will no longer have to understand the mysteries of aging and dying in any deep, existential fashion; we will simply have to pay money to purchase the most up-to-date technologic fixes. Callahan warned that there were two virtually certain results of this shift toward a technologic fix: we will, in the end, fail to solve the problem, and we will go bankrupt trying.

In somewhat the same vein, Kaufman and colleagues describe the biomedicalization of aging in our society as having three key features:

- Life-extending medical care at the end of life and associated medical procedures become routine and expected, rather than consciously chosen.
- The social definitions of "care" and "love" shift to the provision and advocacy of technologies, so that a family of an elderly patient may be seen as insufficiently "loving" unless they are demanding life-extending technology.
- Old age and even death are increasingly defined as treatable and ultimately curable conditions, so that any fatalism or resignation during the waning days of life is a sort of betrayal of a mandatory biomedical optimism.

Kaufman and colleagues then argue that it becomes harder and harder for physicians, nurses, health workers, patients, and families to counter these trends with their individual decisions and care plans. No matter how much ethical powder and shot is expended, actual behavior in health care will conform more and more closely to the newly defined biomedical norm.

On one hand, the arguments presented by Kaufman and colleagues are a helpful reminder of the social background realities against which individual patient care decisions must be made. On the other hand, it is also possible that they have portrayed today's social climate as overly monolithic. To mention just two examples, the powerful social movement toward adoption of complementary and alternative medicine would seem to suggest that the hegemony of biomedicine can be overestimated, and the success of the hospice and palliative care movements would appear to be evidence of the desire of many caregivers, patients, and families for a meaningful alternative to biomedical technology.

In the care of individual patients, Kaufman and colleagues perhaps provide advice on what sorts of questions to ask patients and families who appear to be making irrational end-of-life choices. Inquiry may reveal that they have bought into social or cultural myths about the "cure" of aging and death, indicating the need for helpful counseling to allow them to see the existence of more reasonable and compassionate alternatives. Meanwhile, the entire field of geriatric medicine needs to continue to wrestle with its natural ambivalence over how aging is portrayed to the health care community and the larger society. What is the correct mix between optimism about future technologic and therapeutic progress, and acceptance of human limitations and the continued need for human care and compassion?

References

[1] Emanuel EJ, Emanuel LL. Four models of the physician-patient relationship. JAMA 1992; 267:2221–6.

[2] Kant I. Foundations of the metaphysics of morals: and what is enlightenment? Indianapolis (IN): Bobbs-Merrill; 1959.

[3] Schneider CE. The practice of autonomy. New York: Oxford University Press; 1998.

[4] Fagerlin A, Schneider CE. Enough: the failure of the living will. Hastings Cent Rep 2004; 34(2):30–42.

[5] Lo B. Resolving ethical dilemmas: a guide to clinicians. 2nd edition. Baltimore: Williams and Wilkins; 2000. p. 80–8.

[6] Dworkin R. Life's dominion. New York: Knopf; 1993.

[7] Dresser R. Dworkin on dementia: elegant theory, questionable policy. Hastings Cent Rep 1995;25(6):32–8.

[8] Dresser R, Whitehouse P. The incompetent patient on the slippery slope. Hastings Cent Rep 1994;24(4):6–12.

[9] Kaufman SR, Shim JK, Russ AJ. Revising the biomedicalization of aging: clinical trends and ethical challenges. Gerontologist 2004;44:731–8.

[10] Estes CL, Binney EA. The biomedicalization of aging: dangers and dilemmas. Gerontologist 1989;29:587–97.

[11] Callahan D. Setting limits: medical goals in an aging society. New York: Simon and Schuster; 1987.

ELSEVIER
SAUNDERS

Prim Care Clin Office Pract
32 (2005) 659–669

PRIMARY CARE:
CLINICS IN
OFFICE PRACTICE

Nutrition and Aging

Mary Noel, MPH, PhD, RD*, Mohan Reddy, MD, PhD

Department of Family Practice, College of Human Medicine, Michigan State University, B113 Clinical Center, East Lansing, MI 48824, USA

Consuming a balanced, nutritious diet is important as individuals age [1,2]. However, recommendations made by the office practitioner for such a diet come with the caveat that normal aging is associated with changes in body composition and nutritional requirements. As healthy people age, body fat increases, muscle mass and total body water decrease, and the number of calories necessary to maintain body weight declines. Recommendations and observations on fluid intake are also important because some older adults have decreased thirst. In addition, several medical and neuropsychiatric conditions commonly encountered in the older patient may adversely affect nutrition. Conversely, inadequate nutrition may be associated with a host of poor outcomes for the older adult. Unintended weight loss in particular may herald a terminal downward spiral if the causes of the weight loss are not identified and addressed.

This article describes some aspects of normal aging and their effects on nutritional status, and introduces some of the screening tools used to identify an older adult's nutritional risks. In addition, basic interventions for commonly encountered problems in the office setting are discussed.

Normal aging

The percentage of body fat increases as an individual ages. There is also shift in distribution of body fat, with more deposited in the trunk and less in the extremities. In addition, there is a decrease in muscle and fluid mass, leading to an overall change in body composition that has implications for caloric needs and nutrient requirements and for the distribution and elimination of medications. In general, with usual human aging, there is a decrease in caloric needs of about 2% to 5% for each decade of life and a concomitant decrease in weight. Men usually have their peak weights

* Corresponding author.
E-mail address: noel@msu.edu (M. Noel).

between 55 years of age and the early 60s, whereas women see their peak weights between 65 to 70 years of age [3].

Protein needs do not change substantially. The recommended amount for older adults is 0.8 to 1 g per kilogram of body weight. However, consuming sufficient protein can be difficult for some older adults as appetite wanes, or if finances are limited or cooking skills decline. Vitamins B_{12} and B_6 (pyridoxine), which are found in protein-containing foods, are nutrients that may also be limited in the diets of older adults. In addition to inadequate intake of vitamin B_{12} as a cause of deficiency, older adults may be deficient on the basis of poor absorption because of bacterial overgrowth in the gut as a consequence of a decrease in gastric production of hydrochloric acid that accompanies usual aging or because of abnormalities of intrinsic factors.

Vitamin D and calcium intake require close attention as individuals age because of changes that occur in the skin and kidney. One nutrient that is usually in adequate supply even though intake may not be particularly good is vitamin A. Because of the relative increase in body fat with aging, reserves of this fat-soluble vitamin are usually plentiful. A summary of some physiologic changes of aging and their potential affects on function and nutrition is presented in Table 1.

Assessment tools

As pointed out in the article by Ensberg elsewhere in this issue, a change in appetite or unintended weight loss may reflect impairments in cognitive,

Table 1
Functional and physiologic changes of aging and nutritional needs

Function	Change	Nutrional need
Appetite	↓ Taste ↓ Smell ↓ Visual acuity Dry mouth	1. Social encouragement 2. ↑ Smells & taste of foods 3. Medication review for drugs that ↑ dry mouth; good oral hygiene
Feeding	↓ Shopping and cooking abilities ↓ Dexterity	1. Family and/or community support
Converting food to energy	↓ Basal metabolic rate ↓ GI motility ↑ Bacteria overgrowth of the GI tract ↑ Body fat ↓ Pancreatic enzymes	1. Regular meals 2. Vitamin B_{12} level monitoring 3. Regular PA when possible
Musculoskeletal	↓ Muscle mass ↓ Bone mineralization ↓ Vitamin D conversion by skin and kidney	1. Regular PA 2. Adequate vitamin D and calcium
Elimination	↑ Likelihood of constipation	1. Adequate fiber and fluids

Abbreviations: GI, gastrointestinal; PA, physical activity; ↓, decrease; ↑, increase.
Data from McGee M, Jensen GL. Nutrition in the elderly. J Clin Gastroenterol 2000;30(4):372–80.

physical, or psychosocial functioning. Therefore, tools to help the office-based clinician understand and assess nutrition are essential to providing quality care for the older adult, such as the

- Food pyramid for people over 70 years of age (from Tufts University Center for Nutrition and Aging) [4]
- Determine Your Nutritional Health Checklist (from AAFP, ADA, Council on Aging) (Appendix 1 at the end of this issue)
- DETERMINE Warning Signs (AAFP, ADA, Council on Aging)
- One-day diet record
- Mini Nutrition Assessment [5,6]

The food pyramid for people over 70 years of age (Fig. 1) is a pictorial representation of a healthy diet for older adults. The pyramid emphasizes fruits and vegetables, lean meats and legumes, fiber, and plenty of fluids. Calcium and vitamin D are particularly important. Fluids will help reduce the risk for constipation and the risk for dehydration. Box 1 summarizes the salient features of this pyramid.

Assessment of nutritional problems

Prevention of nutritional problems begins with the assessment of a person's nutritional risk. The Determine Your Nutritional Health Checklist is a useful tool for patients and families to determine nutritional health (Appendix 1 at the end of this issue) [7]. Suggested interventions are provided for each high-risk response on the second sheet of the assessment. Although this assessment tool is not sensitive, it does provide a forum for initiating preliminary discussions about nutrition.

The DETERMINE Warning Signs, which are one component of the materials developed for the Determine Your Nutritional Health initiative and are listed in Box 2, can also be used to assess nutritional risk. Any and all of the factors listed in this mnemonic can place an older adult at nutritional risk. Social and physical changes are most likely to occur when the quality of the diet and overall nutritional status become vulnerable to several insults. Loss of loved ones, inability to shop (perhaps because of having to give up driving), and isolation may decrease the quality and quantity of food eaten. Multiple losses may also be associated with depression and its potential adverse affect on nutrition. For these reasons, most nutritional assessments of the older adult include social dimensions and the traditional dietary intake.

Functional status as a part of nutritional assessment

A person who has difficulty performing the instrumental activities of daily living (IADLs) (Appendix 2 at the end of this issue) is at risk for becoming poorly nourished. For example, difficulty purchasing groceries or

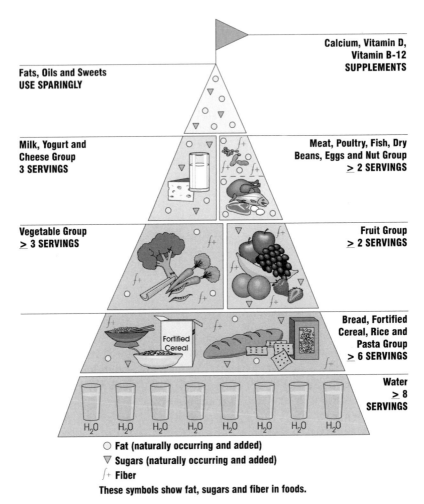

Fig. 1. Guidelines for a healthy diet high in nutrients from Tufts University Center for Nutrition and Aging. (*Data from* Russell RM, Rasmussen H, Lichtenstein AH. Modified food guide pyramid for people over seventy years or age. J Nutr 1999;129:751–3.)

preparing meals may result in poor nutrition unless alternative strategies can be put in place. Other articles in this issue discuss IADLs in more detail and how performance of IADLs can be used to inform an evaluation of the cognitive, physical, or psychosocial impairments that may contribute to poor nutrition [8,9].

Conversely, poor nutrition can lead to functional deficits that may accelerate a decline in the performance of the IADLs. When a physically active person loses weight, up to one third of the weight loss is loss of muscle mass. Muscle loss will be even more pronounced if the person is sedentary. This loss of muscle mass may be associated with fatigue, weakness, or a decline in cognition. If the person who loses weight also becomes

---

Box 1. Summary of healthy diet for people over 70 years of age

Emphasize
- High-fiber–fortified cereals
- Whole grain breads
- Dark green, orange, or yellow vegetables (fresh, frozen, or canned)
- Whole fruits (rather than juices)
- Low-fat dairy products
- Lean meats and fish
- Main dishes of beans, grains, and vegetables

Vary foods in the diet

Drink plenty of fluids

Consider supplements of
- Calcium
- Vitamin D
- Vitamin B_{12}

Low to moderate intake of
- Sugar
- Salt
- Alcohol

Limit foods
- High in refined sugars
- High in saturated fats and cholesterol

Remain physically active

---

bedridden because of medical or neuropsychiatric conditions, pressure ulcers may develop and may be difficult to treat.

Assessment of nutrition in selected disease states

Malnutrition is often not recognized, or when it is, is undertreated in older adults because the nonspecific signs and symptoms may be hard to differentiate from either the consequences of aging or the patient's medical or neuropsychiatric conditions [10–12]. The older adult may look heavy because of a lifetime of being overweight or because of the relative increase in body fat with aging, but he or she may still be poorly nourished. Fatigue and weakness may be related to poor nutrition, as can confusion, decreased immunity, poor tissue healing, and unresponsiveness to treatment. Several chronic diseases are associated with nutritional problems. For example, stroke, Parkinson's disease, and Alzheimer's disease may cause dysphagia. Chronic diseases and the drugs used to treat them may affect the appetite. With respect to drugs and loss of appetite, the usual suspects are digoxin, narcotic analgesics, selective serotonin reuptake inhibitors, and

---

Box 2. DETERMINE Warning Signs

Disease
Eats poorly
Tooth loss/mouth pain
Economic hardship
Reduced social contact
Multiple medicines
Involuntary weight loss/gain
Needs assistance in self care
Elder years above age 80

---

chemotherapeutic agents. However, in any given patient, almost any drug can be associated with decreased appetite. Poor dentition may result in poor intake of meat, fiber, or vegetables.

Unintended weight loss can be another indication of nutritional problems, though the cause may be primarily caused by other things, such as medications, gastrointestinal disease, depression, or a host of other medical or neuropsychiatric conditions. Unintended weight loss seems to shorten life in older adults in contrast to studies in animals that suggest weight loss may lengthen life [13].

Alcohol abuse can be a significant problem in older adults and can cause weight loss and malnutrition. About one third of older alcoholics exhibit problem drinking after the age of 65 years. A history of blackouts, falls, incontinence, malnutrition, vitamin B_{12} or folate deficiency, peripheral neuropathy, myopathy, gout, confusion, or self-neglect can be possible signs of alcohol abuse. Family members or others who shop for the older person may be buying and delivering alcohol along with other groceries. If misuse or abuse is suspected, a screening test should be administered.

Nutrients of concern for all older adults are listed in Table 2 [14].

Adverse effects of nutritional problems

Nutritional deficiencies have been associated with increases in morbidity and mortality, increased rates of infection, and greater use of health care resources. Malnutrition is associated with pressure ulcers, confusion, postural hypotension, infections, and anemia. For the older adult, being underweight is a more important risk factor for death than being overweight. Unintended weight loss in older adults may be overlooked in today's office practice because there is so much emphasis on obesity by health care providers and patients. Problems with eating and feeding also increase caregiver burden [15].

Reviews of the literature suggest that the effectiveness of dietary advice and interventions has been mixed in improving outcomes for older adults, partly because of the varied reasons for illness-related malnutrition [12,16].

Table 2
Nutrients of concern for all older adults

Nutrient	Normal	Indicator		Requirement
Vitamin B$_{12}$	200–900 pg/mL	Shillings Test	↓Abnormal	Deficiency: weekly IM 1000 μg cyanocobalamin
		Methylmalonic acid	↑Abnormal	for 4–8 wk then monthly
		Homocysteine	↑Abnormal	for life: or 1000 to
		Macrocytosis; megaloblastic anemia		2000 μg PO daily for life (RDA is 2–3 μg daily for people who are not deficient.)
Vitamin D				Adequate intake: 51–70 years old 400 IU (10 μg/d); >70 years old 600 IU (15 μg/d)
Calcium		Bone Mineral Density Test		Adequate intake 1200–1500 mg/d

Abbreviations: IM, intramuscularly; RDA, recommended daily allowance; ↓, decrease; ↑, increase.

Physician nutrition assessment tools

Because small amounts of weight loss or gain over time can prove important, it is important to accurately weigh an older patient at every clinical visit. Weight loss should be evaluated if it exceeds 5% of the person's usual weight in 1 month or 10% of the person's usual weight in 3 months.

The one-day food record (items to include in a food record such as presented in Box 3) is a culturally sensitive way for assessing the diet. Clinicians should ask what the person ate and drank yesterday and whether it is representative of the person's usual diet. A person may tell what foods are important and why these foods are important. Clinicians should listen for clues to social issues and the person's abilities, and should note the person's culture, ethnicity, race, or religious group. Clinicians should avoid using a laundry list of typical food preferences, and should determine the pattern of food and fluid consumption.

The Mini Nutritional Assessment [5,6] is a more detailed assessment of the older person's nutritional state (Appendix 1). It uses anthropometric measurements like weight, height, arm and calf circumferences, and weight loss; a general assessment of lifestyle, medication, and mobility; and a dietary history. It can be performed in 10 to 15 minutes and is validated for use in older adults.

Nutritional intervention

Dietary changes should be made cautiously in the older adult, with thoughtful assessment of what the person is currently eating before changes

---

Box 3. Food record of the pattern of food and fluid consumption

- Usual adult weight?
- Recent changes in weight?
- Special diet (type, who prescribed, compliance)?
- Who prepares food?
- Salt added? While cooking? At the table?
- Meals and snacks?
- Fluids during the day, including
  Alcohol?
  Coffee?
  Soft drinks?
- Eats alone? With others?
- Problems affecting intake?
- Who does grocery shopping?

---

are suggested. Even modest restrictions in certain lifelong food consumption patterns may adversely affect the appetite or even the will to eat. Efforts to improve medical conditions with dietary restrictions may convert an already marginal diet to one that is very poor, thereby creating a substantial risk for malnutrition [17].

Management of nutrition and dietary problems

The following steps are useful in managing nutritional problems [2] in the office setting:

- Address and treat early
- Review risk factors
- Treat the treatable
- Prevent further weight loss when possible
- Address issues that fit the problem
- Monitor food intake, meal patterns, quality of food
- Follow preferred meal pattern
- Use supplements judiciously

Avoid restrictive diets if at all possible or recommend only essential restrictions, such as sodium restriction for severe congestive heart failure that has not responded well to other interventions with more liberal sodium intake.

Box 4 lists important potential components of nutritional interventions.

Summary

Nutritional concerns are common among older adults seen in the primary care office. The food pyramid for people over the age of 70 years is a useful

---

Box 4. Nutritional interventions

- Physical activity and exercise, which may enhance appetite and protein intake and increase mobility, strength, and balance
- Alcohol or drug abuse treatment as necessary
- Interdisciplinary team approach as necessary, with referrals to:
  Dentist
  Speech therapist (swallow evaluation)
  Dietitian
  Social services (social, financial services, placement)
  Food service manager and caregivers (for facilitating food intake)
  Psychiatrist (anxiety, depression, psychosis, medication management)
  Occupational therapy (impairment in activities of daily living)
  Physical therapy (pain, mobility)
  Ophthalmologist
  Audiologist
  Other medical specialties
- Community resources for improving services and support in the home
  Family members
  Caregivers
  Meals On Wheels
  Nutrition sites for older adults
  Adult day care programs
  Congregate dining rooms
  Food commodities/food stamps
- Medication
  Review all medications and eliminate any unnecessary medications (no drugs are specifically approved for the treatment of weight loss in older adults)
  Treat depression as appropriate

---

starting point for discussions about what reasonably healthy older adults should be eating and drinking. If there is a decline in the ability to perform IADLs or if there is a decrease in appetite or the discovery of unintended weight loss, careful assessment followed by targeted interventions may improve health outcomes and the quality of life. Restrictive diets are often not well tolerated, especially by frail older adults. Dietary recommendations blending the elements of the pyramid and the essential components of accepted medical nutritional therapy that are most consistent with the patient's lifelong eating patterns are most likely to succeed.

Appendix 1

NESTLÉ NUTRITION SERVICES

Mini Nutritional Assessment
MNA®

Updated Version

Last name:	First name:	Sex:	Date:

Age:	Weight, kg:	Height, cm:	I.D. Number:

Complete the screen by filling in the boxes with the appropriate numbers.
Add the numbers for the screen. If score is 11 or less, continue with the assessment to gain a Malnutrition Indicator Score.

Screening

A Has food intake declined over the past 3 months
due to loss of appetite, digestive problems,
chewing or swallowing difficulties?
0 = severe loss of appetite
1 = moderate loss of appetite
2 = no loss of appetite

B Weight loss during last months
0 = weight loss greater than 3 kg (6.6 lbs)
1 = does not know
2 = weight loss between 1 and 3 kg (2.2 and 6.6 lbs)
3 = no weight loss

C Mobility
0 = bed or chair bound
1 = able to get out of bed/chair but does not go out
2 = goes out

D Has suffered psychological stress or acute
disease in the past 3 months
0 = yes   2 = no

E Neuropsychological problems
0 = severe dementia or depression
1 = mild dementia
2 = no psychological problems

F Body Mass Index (BMI) (weight in kg) / (height in m)²
0 = BMI less than 19
1 = BMI 19 to less than 21
2 = BMI 21 to less than 23
3 = BMI 23 or greater

Screening score (subtotal max. 14 points)

12 points or greater   Normal – not at risk –
no need to complete assessment

11 points or below   Possible malnutrition – continue assessment

Assessment

G Lives independently (not in a nursing home or hospital)
0 = no   1 = yes

H Takes more than 3 prescription drugs per day
0 = yes   1 = no

I Pressure sores or skin ulcers
0 = yes   1 = no

J How many full meals does the patient eat daily?
0 = 1 meal
1 = 2 meals
2 = 3 meals

K Selected consumption markers for protein intake
• At least one serving of dairy products
(milk, cheese, yogurt) per day?   yes ☐ no ☐
• Two or more serving of legumes
or eggs per week?   yes ☐ no ☐
• Meat, fish or poultry every day   yes ☐ no ☐
0.0 = if 0 or 1 yes
0.5 = if 2 yes
1.0 = if 3 yes

L Consumes two or more servings
of fruits or vegetables per day?
0 = no   1 = yes

M How much fluid (water, juice, coffee, tea, milk…)
is consumed per day?
0.0 = less than 3 cups
0.5 = 3 to 5 cups
1.0 = more than 5 cups

N Mode of feeding
0 = unable to eat without assistance
1 = self-fed with some difficulty
2 = self-fed without any problem

O Self view of nutritional status
0 = view self as being malnourished
1 = is uncertain of nutritional state
2 = views self as having no nutritional problem

P In comparison with other people of the same age,
how do they consider their health status?
0.0 = not as good
0.5 = does not know
1.0 = as good
2.0 = better

Q Mid-arm circumference (MAC) in cm
0.0 = MAC less than 21
0.5 = MAC 21 to 22
1.0 = MAC 22 or greater

R Calf circumference (CC) in cm
0 = CC less than 31   1 = CC 31 or greater

Assessment (max. 16 points)

Screening score

Total Assessment (max. 30 points)

Ref   Guigoz Y, Vellas B and Garry PJ. 1994 Mini Nutritional Assessment. A practical assessment tool for grading the nutritional state of elderly patients. *Facts and Research in Gerontology.* Supplement #2 15-59
Rubenstein LZ, Harker J, Guigoz Y and Vellas B. Comprehensive Geriatric Assessment (CGA) and the MNA. An Overview of CGA, Nutritional Assessment, and Development of a Shortened Version of the MNA. In "Mini Nutritional Assessment (MNA): Research and Practice in the Elderly". Vellas B, Garry PJ and Guigoz Y, editors. Nestlé Nutrition Workshop Series. Clinical & Performance Programme, vol 1. Karger, Bâle, in press

® Société des Produits Nestlé S.A., Vevey, Switzerland, Trademark Owners

Malnutrition Indicator Score

17 to 23.5 points	at risk of malnutrition	☐
Less than 17 points	malnourished	☐

From Guigoz Y, Vellas B, Garry PJ. Mini Nutritional Assessment. A practical assessment tool for grading the nutritional state of elderly patients. Facts and Research in Gerontology 1994. Supplement 2:15–59; and Rubenstein LZ, Jarker J, Guigoz Y, et al. Comprehensive Geriatric Assessment (CGA) and the MNA®: an overview of CGA, nutritional assessment, and development of a shortened version of the MNA®. In: Vellas B, Garry PJ, Guigoz Y, editors. Mini Nutritional Assessment (MNA®): Research and practice in the elderly. Nestle Nutrition Workshop Series. Clinical & Performance Programme, vol. 1. Bale (Switzerland): Karger; 1997; with permission ® Société des Produits Nestlé S.A. Vevey, Switzerland, trademark owners.

References

[1] Sullivan DH, Patch GA, Walls RC, et al. Impact of nutrition status on morbidity and mortality in a select population of geriatric rehabilitation patients. Am J Clin Nutr 1990;51: 749–58.

[2] Geriatric Assessment Center of Michigan. Functional assessment of the older adult: incremental assessment. Washington, DC: International Life Sciences Institute; 2003.

[3] Andres R. Body weight and age. In: Brownell KD, Fairburn CG, editors. Eating disorders and obesity: a comprehensive handbook. New York: Guilford Press; 1995.

[4] Russell RM, Rasmussen H, Lichtenstein AH. Modified Food Guide Pyramid for people over seventy years of age. J Nutr 1999;129:751–3.

[5] Guigoz Y, Vellas BJ, Garry PJ. Assessing the nutritional status of the elderly: the Mini Nutritional Assessment as part of the geriatric evaluation. Nutr Rev 1996;54:S59.

[6] Guigoz Y, Lauque S, Vellas BJ. Identifying the elderly at risk for malnutrition. The Mini Nutritional Assessment. Clin Geriatr Med 2002;18(4):737–57.

[7] Huffman GB. Evaluating and treating unintended weight loss in the elderly. Am Fam Phys 2002;65(4):640–50.

[8] Palmer RM. Failure to thrive in the elderly: diagnosis and management. Geriatrics 1990; 45(9):47–55.

[9] Cashman MD. Geriatric malnutrition. Compr Ther 1983;9(7):38–44.

[10] Olsen-Noll CG, Bosworth MF. Anorexia and weight loss in the elderly. Postgrad Med 1989; 85(3):140–4.

[11] Morley JE. Anorexia of aging: physiologic and pathologic. Am J Clin Nutr 1997;66(4): 760–73.

[12] Bales CW, Ritchie CS. Saropenia, weight loss, and nutritional frailty in the elderly. Annu Rev Nutr 2002;22:309–23.

[13] Wilson MM, Morley JE. Physiology of aging, invited review: aging and energy balance. J Appl Physiol 2003;95:1728–36.

[14] Bowman BA, Russell RM. Newer Knowledge in Nutrition. 8th edition. Washington (DC): International Life Sciences Institute; 2001.

[15] Johnson MA, Fischer JG. Eating and appetite: common problems and practical remedies. Generations 2004;28(3):11–7.

[16] Baldwin C, Parsons T, Logan S. Dietary advice for illness-related malnutrition in adults. Cochrane Database Syst Rev 2001;2:CD002008.

[17] Korol DL, Gold PE. Glucose, memory, and aging. Am J Clin Nutr 1998;67(Suppl):S765–71.

ELSEVIER
SAUNDERS

Prim Care Clin Office Pract
32 (2005) 671–682

PRIMARY CARE:
CLINICS IN
OFFICE PRACTICE

Dementia Care: Critical Interactions Among Primary Care Physicians, Patients and Caregivers

Sara B. Holmes, MPH[a],*, Dale Adler, MA, MSW[b]

[a]Michigan Alzheimer's Disease Research Center, Education Core, School of Public Health,
Department of Health Behavior & Health Education, University of Michigan,
1420 Washington Heights, Ann Arbor, MI 48109-2029, USA
[b]14592 Jonathan Harbour Drive, Fort Myers, FL 33908, USA

In the past ten years, enormous progress has been made in understanding and treating Alzheimer's disease (AD) and other dementing illnesses and developing home and community-based support services to assist patients and their families. Today, primary care physicians have greater resources than ever before to provide improved medical care and support services to patients and families facing dementia. The challenges for primary care physicians remain great. They are limited in what they can do by time and reimbursement constraints, lack of knowledge about support services and skepticism about effective medications. In addition, they are faced with how best to communicate and adequately address patient and caregiver concerns throughout the course of the disease. This article reviews the range of interactions and barriers physicians and caregivers face in providing care for patients who have dementia and presents strategies to enhance referral of patients and families to appropriate community support services.

Optimal dementia care: physician, patient and caregiver roles

Most older adults receive their health care solely from their primary care physicians [1]. When symptoms of dementia emerge, patients and their caregivers typically turn first to their primary care physician for answers to

Ms. Holmes work was supported by a grant from the National Institute on Aging of the National Institutes of Health P50-AG08671 (Michigan Alzheimer's Disease Research Center).

* Corresponding author. School of Public Health, University of Michigan, Building II HB & HE, Room 5149, 1420 Washington Heights, Ann Arbor, MI 48103-2023.

E-mail address: holmess@umich.edu (S.B. Holmes).

doi:10.1016/j.pop.2005.07.001
primarycare.theclinics.com

questions about memory loss and obtaining a diagnosis [2]. Therefore, primary care physicians are in a unique position to help patients and family caregivers improve their understanding of the dementia disease process, advise them on managing symptoms as they occur and refer them to appropriate community support services [2].

Often in a primary care setting, the onset and presence of dementia emerges when older patients are treated for other chronic medical conditions such as hypertension, cardiac disease, diabetes, or osteoarthritis. Among the changes in a patient's behavior that may alert the physician to cognitive changes are: missed appointments, non-compliance with medications, frequent telephone calls to the office, missed payments and a family member accompanying the patient to the visit [3]. Unlike the past when dementia patients were often viewed as non-participants in their own care decisions, now that it is possible to establish a diagnosis at an earlier stage, patients are becoming more involved in their own care [2]. Patients, particularly in a primary care setting with a physician they know, often ask to be informed about their diagnosis so they can plan for the future and obtain needed services [4].

Family caregivers also play an important role as a patient's functional and cognitive abilities change by accompanying patients to physician visits and assisting with other activities of daily living. It is important, at this point, for patients to specify relatives or friends that help them and confirm whom they want the physician to contact as future issues emerge.

At some point, when patients who have dementia experience further cognitive decline, they may no longer be a reliable resource for the physician in terms of information exchange and optimal communication. Under these circumstances, the typical physician-patient dyad often expands to a three-way relationship that includes a family caregiver and is referred to as a "health care triad" [2,5]. As dementia progresses, interested caregivers assume greater responsibility for ensuring the person receives appropriate and timely medical care, complies with the treatment plan, undertakes needed safety precautions, and alerts the physician to any changes in the person's condition. Thus, the involvement of family caregivers becomes critical to the physician-patient relationship [6]. In 1999 the American Medical Association recognized the importance of this involvement by calling for a physician/caregiver/patient relationship to meet the needs of patients (who have dementia) and their caregivers [7].

Barriers to optimal dementia care

Physicians and family caregivers, alike have reported a number of barriers in their efforts to provide optimal dementia care.

Physician perspective

A study conducted by Boise [8] with primary care physicians to learn about barriers to adequate dementia diagnosis, found some of their observations were similar to those of caregivers. Reported barriers included physician failure to recognize and respond to symptoms, limited time, perceived lack of need to determine a specific diagnosis and negative attitudes toward the importance of dementia diagnosis and management. Other studies found physicians had difficulty disclosing the diagnosis, giving advice about management and were unaware of support services and how to refer to them. Physicians attending a consensus conference in Michigan in 2001 identified the following additional barriers to implementing dementia practice guidelines: (a) identifying people with dementia opens "Pandora's box", 9b) practice guidelines are difficult to effectively operationalize, 9c) physicians receive inadequate reimbursement for doing a good job, 9d) there are no incentives for quality assessment or follow-up, and 9e) there is a lack of a central (referral) clearinghouse for community resources [9].

Caregiver perspective

Studies have documented that caregivers are often dissatisfied with physician care during the diagnostic process and after the diagnosis is shared with the family [2,10]. Maslow [11] notes that families of people who have AD and related dementias report some physicians do not recognize dementia in their patients and, even if the physician does recognize the condition, he/she may not provide a diagnosis. In a study conducted with one hundred and fifty caregivers, Fortinsky [2] identified four domains of concern regarding their interactions with physicians about dementia care: symptom management; medication management; support service linkage, and emotional support. Participants indicated they were satisfied in general with the medical management of their relative though physician referral to support services were viewed as particularly inadequate. Specifically, caregivers reported they did not receive adequate emotional support or information about symptoms and support services [2].

Family caregivers rely on physicians to provide information about management of dementia symptoms and availability of support services [8]. In fact, caregivers may perceive a physician's referral as having greater legitimacy and be more likely to use services if referred by a physician than someone else [12].

Shared perspective

Physicians, patients and families report it is difficult to locate desired services due to the fragmentation and complexity of accessing services from different systems of care in the community, variance in entrance/exit criteria and capacity to assist people with dementing illnesses. In addition, community and regional differences exist in relation to the scope of available services.

Despite these challenges, studies have begun to identify critical interactions that occur among physicians, patients and caregivers during the course of the disease and suggest interventions to support physicians in managing the ongoing care of patients who have dementia.

Interactions throughout the course of the disease

Numerous studies have confirmed that the needs of patients and families change throughout the course of managing a dementing illness [2]. In early stages of dementia, the major focus of attention among physician, patient and caregiver is to establish the diagnosis and provide patient and caregiver education and support. As dementia symptoms become more persistent and numerous, the interactions focus on symptom management (with or without medication) and use of home and community-based services. In later stages of the disease, considering alternative living facilities and end-of-life care become the focus of family caregivers.

Diagnosis and disclosure

Boise & Connell found that usually patients and families want an accurate and clearly explained diagnosis and guidance from the physician in understanding the course of the illness over time [4]. The article stated: "Specifically caregivers have noted they want physicians to listen to their concerns, devote more time to discussing the diagnosis and what it means, and include the patient even if he or she might not fully understand the implications of the diagnosis." Research has documented that these factors are strongly linked with caregiver satisfaction with the triadic relationship, mentioned earlier.

Boise & Connell emphasize that the disclosure process should be tailored to the manner in which patients and families prefer to have information shared. They found, "For some, this means using a direct approach—having the physician come right out and tell them results of the clinical evaluation for dementia—while others prefer a softer approach. Many physicians and caregivers prefer to focus their discussion on memory problems or safety concerns rather than on the term Alzheimer's disease. Most families eventually want specific information about the diagnosis and its prognosis" [4].

Planning and caregiver support

Primary care physicians are encouraged to discuss advance directives as soon as possible after the diagnosis is disclosed, so patients can be involved to the greatest extent possible. Patients and families should also be urged to begin advance planning with regard to durable power of attorney and financial management [13].

As mentioned earlier, as the patient becomes increasingly impaired, the physician depends on the family caregiver to ensure that the patient receives good medical care and follows the physician's instructions. In the AMA's 1999 guide, physicians are encouraged to assess the needs of family caregivers, ask how they are coping, provide information about what they can expect in the future, and provide resources that can reduce caregiver stress, anxiety, depression and sleep deprivation. In addition, Glasser and Miller recommend physicians build in brief periods of time to ask the caregiver how she/he is doing and coping [14]. Also, if the caregiver is the physician's patient, the physician can assess their caregiver status as part of their regular exam. Physicians suggest in Connell's study (2004) that they should have increased time available to spend with patients and their caregivers [10]. This supports a recommendation made earlier by the Council on Scientific Affairs of the American Medical Association to reimburse physicians for time spent educating and counseling caregivers [15].

Referral and use of community resources

Following a diagnosis, physicians are in a unique position to refer patients and families to community organizations that offer educational information on the progression and management of dementia symptoms and direct support services (ie, counseling, in-home respite, and adult day services). The importance of these services cannot be overestimated. Numerous studies have shown significantly improved patient and caregiver outcomes when caregiver needs are assessed and education or counseling provided [16]. A study by Mittleman and colleagues showed that comprehensive support and counseling for spouse-caregivers delayed nursing home placement of patients who have mild to moderate Alzheimer's disease [17]. Another study showed that counseling by telephone assisted spouse caregivers in feeling more competent and knowledgeable about Alzheimer's disease and more independent in making caregiving decisions [18].

Physicians encounter and report challenges to providing up-to-date information and referral to services especially in rural areas where services might be scarce [10]. In an earlier study by Fortinsky, physician survey results indicated that unfamiliarity with community services was the most common barrier to ongoing management of patients who have dementia [19]. Most physicians were interested, however, in linking with community services and willing to share the ongoing management of patients who have dementia and families with community services. Perhaps the most significant obstacle to referral for community support services is the lack of time available to physicians to learn about and remain apprised of specific available resources. The AMA Guide for Primary Care Physicians on the Diagnosis, Management and Treatment of Dementia recommends that an office staff member be assigned to develop expertise on community resources and become the primary link between patients, families and the community resources they need [7].

Additional strategies to assist physicians in sharing the ongoing management of patients and families include: "referral to social service agencies or support organizations, including the Alzheimer's Association's

Safe Return Program for people who may wander" and "referral to support organizations for educational materials on community resources, support groups, legal and financial issues, respite care and future care needs and options" [13]. Box 1 provides information about key resources nationally and locally.

Box 2 describes the broad array of services frequently used by patients and families. Families can be encouraged to access printed and online resources about dementing illnesses and strategies that may help them cope with demands and role changes they will encounter in caring for someone who has dementia. These include: newsletters, pamphlets, booklets and information on the websites of the resources listed in Box 1.

There are many considerations in successfully linking patients and families to home-based and community support services to supplement

---

Box 1. Resources for information about Alzheimer's disease and other dementing illnesses, community resources and support services

Alzheimer's Association: Source of valuable information about all aspects of care for people who have dementia and their families. More than 80 chapters nationwide provide care consultation, support groups, 24/7 support line services, education and safe return programs. For a local chapter contact: (800) 337-3827. Website: http://www.alz.org

Area Agencies on Aging (AAA): Local AAAs offer information and assistance with locating a range of elder care services. These include: care management services, home-delivered and congregate meals, homemaker and personal care services. Contact Eldercare Locator: (800) 677-1116. Website: http://www.aoa.dhhs.gov

Alzheimer's Disease Education and Referral (ADEAR) Center: A service of the National Institute on Aging to compile, archive and disseminate information concerning Alzheimer's disease for health professionals, people who have AD and their families, and the public. Specialists are available to answer specific questions about AD, send free publications, refer to local supportive services, and offer Spanish language resources and clinical trials information. Telephone: (800) 438-4380. Website: http://www.alzheimers.org

Family Caregiver Alliance: A national organization dedicated to working with caregivers. They provide fact sheets, research updates and an e-mail-based support group. Telephone: (415) 434-3388. Website: http://www.caregiver.org

Box 2. Frequently used home and community-based support services

In-Home resources
Home health care
Provides medical assistance (skilled nursing, rehabilitation
   therapy, home health aides) to older persons in their homes.
   This is doctor-prescribed and the attending physician needs
   to be involved directly in order for this type of care to be
   covered under Medicare or private insurance.
Personal care services
Includes bathing and dressing and are not Medicare-reimbursed.
   They are available privately or through home health agencies.
Homemaking/chore services
Includes laundry, shopping, housecleaning and are not
   Medicare-reimbursed.
In-home respite care:
Provided in the home by professional caregivers or trained
   volunteers; they can be employed privately or through an
   agency and either private, non-profit or government funded.
   Services may include: companionship, personal care,
   homemaking, or skilled care.

Community-based resources
Care management
Provides help by a professional in coordinating services for
   persons with dementia and their families.
Support groups
Help caregiver cope and gather information. Patients may
   participate in the early stages.
Adult day services
Offer group respite care that is provided outside the home and
   designed to support the strengths, abilities, and independence
   of each participant.
Residential/overnight respite care
Residential facilities may allow the person who has dementia to
   stay overnight, for a few days, or a few weeks. Many hospitals
   and nursing home have specialized units for this purpose.
For additional information about these services or finding local
   offices: Alzheimer's Association telephone: (800) 337-3827; or
   Area Agencies on Aging (AAA), Eldercare Locator, telephone
   (800) 677-1116.

support provided by the patient's informal network of families, friends and neighbors. A variety of issues may influence the timing and receptivity of family caregivers to physician recommendations. Among these include: (1) the degree of confidence, trust and credibility established in the triadic relationship; (2) functional status of both the patient and caregiver; (3) cultural norms and factors related to a family's beliefs and attitudes about its responsibilities, decision-makers and involving outsiders; (4) awareness by the physician and family, alike about the types and scope of available community resources, eligibility criteria, and who to contact to find out; (5) the physician's assessment of the family's readiness to consider alternative support strategies; and (6) perceptions about the responsiveness, quality and appropriateness of available services [20].

Palliative and end-of-life care

As patients approach the late stages of AD or other dementing illnesses, physicians have the difficult task of helping the family make decisions about terminal care. Early discussions about "do not resuscitate" orders, the use of antibiotics for infections, and the initiation of tube feeding will help the physician understand the beliefs and preferences of the patient and family [13]. Optimal end-of-life care for individuals who have dementia care occurs when family members can develop a plan well ahead of time that reduces the likelihood of invasive and unnecessary medical interventions. Hospice care can be invaluable for the family of a patient who has end-stage Alzheimer's disease. Box 3 provides the hospice eligibility criteria for patients who have dementia.

Emerging strategies to effectively link patients and families with services

The final section describes three service models to support physicians in managing ongoing care of patients who have dementia: An Alzheimer's Service Coordination Program, Chronic Care Network for Alzheimer's Disease and Academic Detailing Community Resource Teams. Based on the research finding that most physicians are willing to share the ongoing care of patients who have dementia, a service model was developed and piloted in Cleveland (1996–1998) to link primary care physicians with a community organization that specializes in dementia education and support (in this case, a local Alzheimer's Chapter) [21]. The Alzheimer's Service Coordination Program was designed to have physicians initiate the program by asking patients and families at the time of diagnosis if they were interested in referral to the local Alzheimer's chapter for educational and counseling services. If the patient and family sign a consent form, a referral is sent to the chapter listing the major concerns the family expressed to the physician. This allows the Chapter to initiate contact with the family to address their concerns. After the six-month pilot project, 44 caregivers reported

---

Box 3. Hospice eligibility for people who have dementia

Alzheimer's disease and other dementias have both a chronic and terminal stage. It is during the terminal stage when hospice may be sought.

A person enters this terminal phase when they show all of these signs:

- unable to walk without assistance
- unable to dress themselves
- need help bathing and/or grooming
- unable to control bladder and bowel
- unable to converse or communicate verbally

A person must also show at least *one* of the following within the last year to be eligible:

- serious lung or kidney infection
- sepsis (or blood poisoning)
- severe open bedsores or pressure ulcers
- persistent fever, even after antibiotics
- consistent inability to take food/fluids, or profound nutritional impairment

Once the above criteria are met, a physician must certify that the person has a limited life expectance of six months or less, or as long as the disease runs its normal course.

COST

All Medicare and Medicaid Part A plans have a hospice benefit that will pay for hospice medical and counseling services.

However, hospice does *not* pay for room and board. Most private insurance providers include a hospice benefit but plans differ and families should check with their individual provider.

———

Data from Local Medical Review Policy Guidelines for Persons with Advanced Dementia.

---

statistically significant increases in self-efficacy in managing dementia symptoms and using community resources. In addition, the 29 participating physicians and 62 participating caregivers reported satisfaction with the program [2]. Currently, adaptations of this program, called "positive referral service" are being initiated between physician offices and local Alzheimer's chapters throughout the country [21].

Another project designed to achieve multiple goals in supporting family caregivers is a joint project of the Alzheimer's Association and the National Chronic Care Consortium called: Chronic Care Networks for Alzheimer's Disease (CCN/AD). The CCN/AD Initiative was a six-year demonstration project that implemented a model of dementia care that was designed to (a) improve the identification of possible dementia in health care settings; (b) adopt a practical model of dementia assessment; (c) improve coordination between medical care and supportive services through the development of partnerships between health care providers and Alzheimer's Association chapters and (d) introduce systems change that would guide the overall care of individuals, not just their dementia. The multi-site initiative was implemented in six communities under various types of health care systems and arrangements. The variety of arrangements among the participating health systems provided an opportunity to see how changes in dementia care practices can occur within different types of networks. The CCN/AD Model of Care included four components:

- Identification of possible dementia through a variety of provider training modalities and use of a family questionnaire to identify changes in activities of daily living (ADL) performance.
- List of dementia assessment procedures, of which some or all could be implemented and used by physicians, nurses and others.
- Use of care management blue prints, a source of ideas which sites could use to develop their own protocols for assessment and possible interventions in six domains.
- Provision of information and support for family caregivers, which uses a grid with objectives to be achieved for families in six phases of caregiving: (1) prediagnostic, (2) diagnostic, (3) role change, (4) chronic caregiving, (5) transition to alternative care, and (6) end of life. See caregiver support grid shown in Table 1.

The caregiver support grid can be used to identify the types of material and services caregivers may need at each phase and where there might be gaps in materials and services. Because the grid places an emphasis on the caregiver's tasks and challenges, it is more likely that the information and programs provided to families will meet their needs [11]. Similar to a referral method piloted through the Alzheimer's Service Coordination Program, the CCN/ AD Initiative found it helpful for health care providers to use and fax referral consent forms to participating Alzheimer's Association offices. This allowed chapters to initiate contact with enrollees and their families and facilitate early linkage with information and non-medical support services [22].

A third strategy that will be piloted in summer 2005 to strengthen the link between physician offices and local community services is called "academic detailing community resource teams." In a program conducted by the Primary Care Dementia Leaders Network in Michigan, a team composed of a retired physician, a representative from the local Alzheimer's Chapter and the local AAA will schedule brief visits with interested physician practices in their area. Using a common marketing strategy found in health care, the visit is designed to introduce physicians and their staff to local community support services, describe how the services help patients who have dementia and their families and provide educational materials targeted to

Table 1
Caregiver support grid diagnostic phase

	Objective	Program(s)*	Provided by	Appropriate materials*
1.**	Obtain an accurate diagnosis. Know how to get a second opinion if necessary.			
2.	Understand how the diagnosis was made.			
3.	Know how to approach the patient with news.			
4.**	Know what possible treatments exist.			
5.	Begin to accept the diagnosis and patient's limitations.			
6.**	Understand the need for proactive planning, including financial, legal, and care plans.			
7.	Seek out supportive services is needed (early-stage support groups, education sessions, etc.).			

* All programs and materials should be adapted to meet the needs of families with different ethnic, cultural, and economic backgrounds and different primary languages.
** These objectives were identified as most important by site-level project staff and were used for evaluation purposes.
(*Data from* National Chronic Care Consortium and the Alzheimer's Association)

professionals, patients and families about support services. Results of the pilot phase of the project will be available in winter, 2006.

References

[1] Ganguli M, Rodriguez E, Mulsant B, et al. Detection and management of cognitive impairment in primary care: The Steel Valley Seniors Survey. J Am Geriatr Soc 2004;52: 668–75.
[2] Fortinsky RH. Health care triads and dementia care: integrative framework and future direction. Aging Ment Health 2001;5:S35–48.
[3] Lawhone L, Weaver D, Walsh K. Michigan Primary Care Dementia Network. Triggers, Academic Detailing Training Manual. East Lansing (MI): Geriatric Education Center of Michigan; 2005.
[4] Boise L, Connell CM. Aging and Geriatrics 2005; In press.
[5] Haug MR. Elderly patients, caregivers, and physicians: Theory and research on health care triads. J Health Soc Behav 1994;35:1–12.
[6] Beisecker AE, Chrisman SK, Wright LJ. Perceptions of family caregivers of persons with Alzheimer's disease: Communication with physicians. Am J Alzheimer's Dis Other Demen 1997;12:73–83.
[7] American Medical Association. In: Gattman R, Seleski M, editors. Diagnosis, management and treatment of dementia: A practical guide for physicians. Chicago: American Medical Association; 1999.

[8] Boise L, Camicioli R, Morgan D, et al. Diagnosing dementia: perspectives of primary care physicians. Gerontologist 1999;39:457–64.

[9] Michigan Primary Care Dementia Network. Barriers to best primary care practices in dementia. Presented at the First Annual Meeting of Michigan Primary Care Network. Midland, Michigan, December 1, 2001.

[10] Connell CM, Boise L, Stuckey JC, et al. Attitudes toward the diagnosis and disclosure of dementia among family caregivers and primary care physicians. Gerontologist 2004;44: 500–7.

[11] Maslow K, Selstad J. Chronic care networks for Alzheimer's disease: approaches for involving and supporting family caregivers in an innovative model of dementia care. Alzheimer's Care Quarterly 2001;2:33–46.

[12] Maslow K. Linking persons with dementia to appropriate services: summary of an OTA study. Pride Inst J Long Term Home Health Care 1990;9:42–50.

[13] Cummings J, Frank J, Cherry D, et al. Guidelines for managing Alzheimer's disease: Part II. treatment. Am Fam Physician 2002;65:2525–34.

[14] Glasser M, Miller B. Caregiver and physician perspectives of medical encounters involving dementia patients. Am J Alzheimer's Dis Other Demen 1998;13:70–9.

[15] Council on Scientific Affairs. Physicians and family caregiver: A model for partnership. JAMA 1993;269:1282–4.

[16] Chow TW, Maclean CH. Quality indicators for dementia in vulnerable community-dwelling and hospitalized elders. Ann Intern Med 2001;35:668–76.

[17] Mittleman MS, Ferris SH, Shulman E, et al. A family intervention to delay nursing home placement of patients with Alzheimer's disease: A randomized controlled trial. JAMA 1996; 276:1725–31.

[18] Chiverton P, Caine ED. Education to assist spouses in coping with Alzheimer's disease: A controlled trial. Journal of American Geriatrics Society 1989;37:593–8.

[19] Fortinsky RH. How linked are physicians to community support services for their patients with dementia? J Appl Gerontol 1998;17:480–98.

[20] Thakur NM, Perkel RL. Prevention in adulthood: forging a doctor-patient partnership. Primary Care Clinic Office Practice 2002;29:571–82.

[21] Fortinsky RH, Unson CG, Garcia RI. Helping family caregivers by linking primary care physicians with community-based dementia care services. Dementia 2002;1:227–40.

[22] Maslow K. Changing dementia care practice in various healthcare settings. Presented at the Third Annual Meeting of the Michigan Primary Care Dementia Network. East Lansing, Michigan, October 25, 2003.

ELSEVIER
SAUNDERS

Prim Care Clin Office Pract
32 (2005) 683–697

PRIMARY CARE:
CLINICS IN
OFFICE PRACTICE

The Slippery Slope: Reducing Fall Risk in Older Adults

Francis A. Komara, DO

*Michigan State University, College of Osteopathic Medicine, B211 West Fee Hall,
East Lansing, MI 48824, USA*

Evaluating and managing falls in older adults are important tasks for the office-based primary care provider. Falls may result in serious injuries, even death. But perhaps just as important, fear of falling may lead to reduced mobility, deconditioning, dependencies, social isolation, and diminished quality of life. A major difficulty in the evaluation of the older adult who falls is that by the time a fall has occurred, significant deficits in physical function already may be present. In addition, a fall is often the consequence of several intrinsic, extrinsic, or situational risk factors suggesting that interventions to reduce the chances of future falls and associated injuries will require multifaceted interventions.

A fall is defined as failure to maintain an appropriate lying, sitting, or standing position, resulting in an individual's abrupt, undesired relocation to the ground [1]. Falls are a leading cause of nonfatal injuries in adults 65 years of age and over, with people over 75 years of age more prone to long-term disability and death than those in younger age groups. Of all medical expenditures for adults over 65 years of age, 6% are accounted for by fall injury [2].

This article focuses on ways to identify risk factors before a fall occurs and discusses approaches to implementing interventions that reduce fall risk factors and minimize the consequences of falls that do occur. As has been suggested in the article by Ensberg elsewhere in this issue, by simply observing the patient arising from the chair in the waiting room, walking to the examination room, and getting onto the examination table, staff members may be able to identify someone who should undergo further evaluation.

E-mail address: komaraf@msu.edu

Epidemiology of falls and injuries

Fig. 1 depicts the distribution of fatal and nonfatal injuries by age and mechanism of injury. The contribution of falls to fatal injuries escalates from no more than 6% in the under 65-year age groups to 36% for those over 65 years of age. For nonfatal injuries, the differences are not as dramatic, with falls accounting for 16% to 36% of injuries in the group under the age of 65 years compared with 63% for people over the age 65 years [3].

The distribution of types of injuries resulting from falls for people over the age of 65 years is as follows: (1) 19.1% of the injuries among men are fractures (29.5% for women), (2) 21.7% of the injuries among men are contusions or abrasions (24.2% for women), and (3) 23.4% of the injuries among men are lacerations or puncture wounds (15.1% for women) [3]. Unintentional injuries, including falls, were the seventh leading cause of death in the 65-years-and-over age group [4].

Prospective studies of community-dwelling older persons suggest that 30% to 60% of them fall each year with a mean fall rate of 0.7 falls per year. Forty-three percent of institutionalized older persons fall each year, with a fall rate of 1.6 falls per bed in nursing facilities and 1.4 falls per bed in hospital settings [5]. Of concern is that 50% of all fractures that occur in institutionalized older persons are hip fractures and that 25% of those who have a hip fracture in an institution die within a year following the hip fracture. Common characteristics of falls with fractures are that they occur during the day, in the bedroom, during ambulation, or in association with a wet floor [6]. Recurrent or frequent fallers are defined as people who fall at least three times per month. Many studies have supported the observation that decreased use of restraints has not been associated with an increase in fall or injury rate.

A fall or the fear of falling in the older adult should trigger the office-based clinician to think about the possibility of functional decline. In addition, it is important to consider that the person who falls or who fears falling may not be experiencing mild or early functional deficits but may already be in the midst of a progressive deterioration of physical function. In 1986, Tinetti [7] cited a report from the Canadian Task Force on the Periodic Health Examination noting the decline in mobility with aging, and concluded that several factors associated with the chronic diseases and disabilities common among older adults contribute to an increased risk for falling, especially for patients over the age of 75 years. Tinetti emphasized that preservation of abilities should be emphasized over diagnosis because it is the decline in abilities that makes the older person vulnerable.

Considering the continuum of activity ranging from mobility to falls to immobility, clinicians may be waiting too long to identify patients who have a decline in physical conditioning or mobility if actions are taken only after a fall has occurred. By simply asking at each visit about the patient's fear of

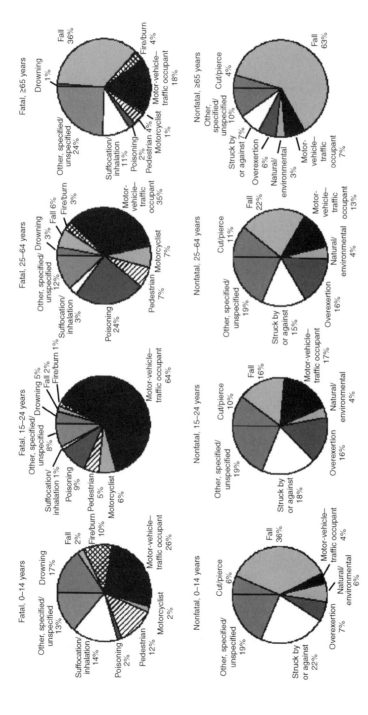

Fig. 1. Fatal and nonfatal injuries by age and mechanism of injury. *(From* Vyrostek SB, Annest JL, Ryan GW. Surveillance for fatal and nonfatal injuries–United States, 2001. MMWR Surveill Summ 2004;53(7):1–57; with permission.)

falling or about changes in balance and gait, office-based clinicians may be able to address functional declines before the fall.

A search for risk factors should complement these questions so that as many as possible can be eliminated or reduced.

Risk factors for falls

Multiple studies have determined important risk factors for falling in older adults. Muscle weakness, previous falls, dependency in any activities of daily living (ADL) or instrumental activities of daily living (IADL), balance and gait disorders, use of an assistive device, vision deficit, arthritis, depression, and impaired cognition all contribute to higher fall risk [2]. Box 1 lists the mean relative risk ratio (RR) and odds ratio (OR) of risk factors for falls that were determined from 16 studies.

Risk factors for a fall with a serious injury include advanced age, cognitive impairment, female gender, the presence of at least two chronic conditions, low body mass index, and impaired balance and gait [8]. Cognitive impairment may foster injury because of a diminished protective response or impaired judgment, placing the individual in unsafe situations. Medication use has also been associated with increased fall risk in older persons in several studies, especially for people on three or more medications [5]. Specific medications associated with an increase in the risk for falls are psychotropic drugs, including neuroleptics, antidepressants (especially the tricyclics), sedative/hypnotics, and benzodiazepines [9]. A meta-analysis of cardiac and analgesic drugs found an association between falls and the use of diuretics, digoxin, and type IA antiarrhythmics [10].

The more risk factors present, the greater the risk for falling. Tinetti and colleagues [11] reported that in older persons living in the community, the risk for falling increased with the number of risk factors, from 8% who had

---

Box 1. Mean RR or OR of risk factors for falls from 16 studies

- Muscle weakness: 4.4
- History of falls: 3.0
- Gait or balance deficit: 2.9
- Use of assistive device: 2.6
- Visual deficit: 2.5
- Arthritis: 2.4
- Depression: 2.2
- Cognitive impairment: 1.8
- Age over 80 years: 1.7

Data from AGS Panel on Falls Prevention. Guideline for the prevention of falls in older persons. J Am Geriatr Soc 2001;49(5):664–72.

no risk factors to 19% who had one risk factor, up to 78% who had four or more risk factors. Furthermore, 10% of falls occur during an acute illness.

The causes of falls from 12 studies were reviewed by Rubenstein and Josephson [5] with the leading causes being an accident or environmentally related event (31%); gait and balance disorders (17%); dizziness (13%); drop attack (9%); confusion (5%); postural hypotension (3%); and visual disorder (2%). Accidental falls occurred more frequently in the home, involving environmental hazards such as wet floors and poor lighting. Ten percent of falls occur on stairs, with more falls during descent than ascent and greater risk for falls associated with the first and last steps. Curbs, steps, and uneven pavement are common obstacles outdoors [12]. Stroke, Parkinson's disease, and arthritis are common diseases associated with gait and balance problems.

The multifactorial nature of falls and fall-related injuries has been demonstrated. Equally important is the observation that a fall is often the cumulative result of several risk factors, each with a small relative risk [7]. Therefore, once the office-based clinician has identified a patient who is concerned about falling, whether a fall has occurred or not, a systematic evaluation to identify risk factors for falls should be initiated. In addition, an incremental assessment of overall functional status is warranted. Delaying evaluation until after the fall has occurred could be life-threatening for the patient given the outcomes for fall-associated hip fractures.

The incremental functional assessment approach is described in detail in the article by Ensberg elsewhere in this issue, but several points should be emphasized here. Evaluation of the older adult should routinely include questions about falls or concern about falling. A review of the patient's ability to perform ADLs and IADLs should be triggered anytime a fall occurs or the person expresses concern about falling or reports a change in balance or gait. Review of systems should focus on memory, vision, hearing, and bowel and bladder function. The physical exam should include cognitive and mood screens; simple tests for vision and hearing; blood pressure readings in supine, sitting, and standing positions; and balance, gait, and mobility testing. Rubenstein and colleagues [13] studied the quality of care that community-based physicians in a managed care organization provided to vulnerable older persons who had fallen or reported instability. They found that evaluation and management were not consistent with existing guidelines, including some of the elements just described. For example, only 15% of falls and 6% of mobility problems were documented in the history. In the physical examination of fallers, 28% did undergo a neurologic examination and 25% were tested for vision, but only 6% had orthostatic blood pressures measured and only 7% examined for gait and balance.

In summary, any positive response to periodic questions about falls, fear of falling, or concerns about balance or gait should prompt a more in-depth evaluation looking for as many risk factors as possible (eg, muscle weakness, advanced age, prior falls, multiple medications, vision or hearing deficits). Experience shows that as age increases from 65 years, the number of falls increases. Therefore, whether or not a fall has yet to occur, the patient should be queried at regular intervals. Finally, when a fall does occur, it is unlikely that a single risk factor will be at play; the fall is likely to be multifactorial requiring a multifaceted set of interventions. It is probably impossible to prevent all falls; the goals should be to eliminate or reduce as many risk factors as possible and to minimize the complications from falls that do occur.

Clinical approach

The focus of the evaluation is to identify risk factors with appropriate screens. Interventions can then be targeted to address each identified risk factor. The overall health of each individual should be considered, including medical and surgical status, predicted response to rehabilitation and conditioning, and possible outcomes with environmental modifications. The diagram described in Ensberg's article that depicts the intersection of circles representing cognitive, physical, psychosocial, and spiritual domains within the person's environmental setting is especially appropriate as it pertains to falls. Even when providers documented falls in the history (85%), appropriate physical examination was documented only 20% of the time [13]. The patient who has a hip fracture, contusion of the face, or some other obvious injury will likely be evaluated and treated promptly. For the person who has a noninjurious fall or one who fears falling or is concerned about balance or gait, evaluation of all aspects of the fall and the fall risk assessment may be too time-consuming to complete during a single visit. Many patients can be evaluated incrementally to identify all of the factors involved.

Box 2 provides a checklist of the evaluations (the ten S's) that can be performed incrementally over time.

Specific risk factor screens that may be performed include the Mini-Cog or mini-mental status examination (MMSE) (Appendix 3c at the end of this issue) for cognition; blood pressure evaluation in supine, sitting, and standing positions; and evaluation of arm strength by having the patient lift a book over the head or, as an initial evaluation, just raise the hands over the head. Leg strength is examined by having the person assume a standing position from a chair without pushing off of the arms and by standing up on tiptoe while being stabilized behind a standard chair. Balance can be evaluated by having the patient stand on one leg or perform a tandem walk. Always stand by the patient during these tests in case he or she is unable to maintain balance. Gait should be assessed by having the patient walk 10 feet, and then turn and walk back. Attention should be given to observing the patient on the turn to see if there is a problem maintaining balance. Again, the patient should be spotted during these maneuvers. Medications should be reviewed on each office visit to identify those that are associated

---

Box 2. The ten S's

Structure
  Anatomy
  Arthritis (spine, hips, knees, ankles, feet)
  Range of motion
Stride
  Step length, gait, symmetry, stride length, shuffle
Speed
Sepsis
  Infection
Strength
  Upper and lower extremities
Sway
  Balance, postural reflexes
Surface
  Environment: wetness, ice, snow
  Even or uneven flooring, pavement, or ground
  Slippery floors
  Obstacles: throw rugs, extension cords, clutter
Shoes
  Heels, slippery or tacky sole material, shoe fit
Sensorium
  Delirium, depression, dementia
  Medications: drug interactions, polypharmacy (more than
    three or four drugs)
  Fear of falling
Sight
  Visual acuity, cataracts, glaucoma

---

with increased fall risk to be sure that each is still necessary, to inquire about possible side effects, and to consider drug–drug interactions.

Comments about specific screening

Orthostatic blood pressure changes

Blood pressure determination in multiple positions is probably underused. In addition, blood pressure is not always measured according to standard protocol. Blood pressure should not be taken through clothing. It should be measured in the supine, sitting, and standing positions, with the supine reading taken after the patient has been supine at least 5 minutes, and the sitting and standing blood pressures taken at 1 minute and 3 minutes. This practice will identify changes in pressure that are immediate or late [14].

Performance screens

The performance criteria can be screened by using several tools that are readily available. The Timed Get Up and Go Test (Appendix 4a at the end of this issue) has the patient arise from a standard chair without using the hands, walk 10 feet to a line on the floor, turn, return to the chair, and then sit down. The test is timed and persons who require more than 10 seconds for this test may have physical limitations that predispose to falls. Normal time is 7 to 10 seconds. Patients who perform the test in less than 20 seconds still have independent mobility, but as the time increases above 20 seconds, further evaluation will be necessary to assess the risk for falls [15]. Patients who have difficulty rising from the chair may have quadriceps muscle weakness.

Another commonly used mobility screen is the Performance-Oriented Mobility Assessment by Tinetti [7]. The test includes several maneuvers to assess balance (Table 1) and gait (Table 2) that simulate activities the patient will encounter during typical daily activities.

Medication assessment

Evaluation of the patient's medications should occur regularly. Note the total number, class, and dosage. Consider the continued need for each medication and its possible side effects and interactions with other medications, including prescription and over-the-counter. Examples of over-the-counter medications that may be overlooked are sleep aids such as acetaminophen with diphenhydramine. Patients may take such preparations nightly believing them to be safe because they are available without a prescription. They may, however, be a prime contributor to falls because of their risk for orthostatic hypotension. As described earlier, specific classes of medications that have been implicated as potential contributors to falls are diuretics, digoxin, type IA antiarrhythmics, nitrates, and psychoactive medications, including neuroleptics and antidepressants, especially tricyclic antidepressants. Consulting a pharmacist or computer program to identify adverse drug reactions or drug–drug interactions can be helpful when conducting these drug regimen reviews.

Intervention

Once screening tests and other evaluations have identified specific risk factors, an individualized multifaceted treatment plan can be devised. If the patient is found to have altered cognition, such as delirium or dementia (Appendices 3d,e at the end of this issue), then the underlying causes of the delirium should be addressed or specific dementia interventions, including behavioral strategies, can be initiated. Patients who are found to be depressed should be treated with nonpharmacologic and pharmacologic therapy, taking care that the drugs used to treat depression do not increase fall risk.

Table 1
Performance-oriented assessment of balance: response

Maneuver	Normal	Adaptive	Abnormal
Sitting balance	Steady, stable	Holds onto chair	Leans, slides down
Arising from chair	Able to rise without arms	Uses arms	Multiple attempts needed
Immediate standing balance (3–5 s)	Steady without walking aid	Steady with aid	Unsteady
Standing balance	Steady without holding object	Steady but can't put feet together	Unsteady
Balance with eyes closed	Steady without holding object	Steady with feet apart	Unsteady
Turning balance	No grabbing, steps continuous	Steps discontinuous	Unsteady
Sternal nudge, feet together	Steady	Needs to move feet to maintain balance	Begins to fall
Neck turning	Able to turn head, look at ceiling, no stagger	Decreased ability to turn and extend neck, no stagger	Unsteady
One leg standing balance	Able to stand 5 s without support		Unable
Back extension	Good extension	Attempts extension, decreased range of motion	No extension, staggers
Reaching up	Able to take down object without support	Able to retrieve object with support	Unsteady
Bending down	Able to bend without support	Able to bend with support	Unable, unsteady
Sitting down	Able to sit in one movement	Needs arms to guide sitting	Falls into chair, misjudges distance

Data from Tinetti ME. Performance-oriented assessment of mobility problems in elderly patients. J Am Geriatr Soc 1986;34(2):119–26.

If orthostatic hypotension is identified, medication should be adjusted. Other strategies include elevating the head of the bed, use of support stockings, minimizing salt restriction, and sitting at the side of the bed for 5 minutes before arising. An exercise program can be beneficial in normalizing blood pressure response.

Inactivity and lack of physical exercise are major contributors to fall risk, and the best approach to improving muscle strength is exercise. The use of resistance exercises can benefit arm and leg strength. The Centers for Disease Control and Prevention recommends strength or resistance training for adults over the age of 65 years. Resistance training results in increased muscular strength and improved endurance and bone density. Resistance exercises can reduce the risk for falls and encourage independent living [16]. One of the national health objectives of the Healthy People 2010 program by the US Department of Health and Human Services is to increase to 30%

Table 2
Performance-oriented assessment of gait: observation

Component	Normal	Abnormal
Initiation of gait	Begins walking immediately, smooth motion	Hesitates, not fluid
Step height	Swing foot clears floor by 1–2 inches	Swing foot not raised off floor or too high >1–2 inches
Step length	At least foot length between stance toe and swing heel	Length less than normal
Step symmetry	Step length same bilaterally	Step length varies
Step continuity	Begins raising heel of one foot as heel of other foot touches the floor (heel strike)	Places entire foot on floor before raising the other foot
Path deviation	Foot follows close to straight line with advance	Foot deviates from side to side
Trunk stability	Trunk without sway, knees and back not flexed, arms not abducted	Any sway, knee or back flexion, abduction of arms
Walk stance	Feet almost touch as they pass each other	Feet apart while stepping
Turning while walking	No stagger, continuous	Stagger, stops with turn, not continuous

Data from Tinetti ME. Performance-oriented assessment of mobility problems in elderly patients. J Am Geriatr Soc 1986;34(2):119–126.

the percentage of adults who perform two or more days per week of physical activity that enhances muscle strength and endurance [16]. At present, only 12% of adults aged 65 to 74 years and 10% of those aged 75 years and older meet the strength training recommendation of this objective. In addition, when older adults were asked to self-categorize leisure physical activity level, only 24.7% categorized themselves as active, 14% as insufficiently active, and 4% as inactive [15]. In this survey, "active" was defined as moderate physical activity for 5 or more days per week for 30 or more minutes per session or 3 or more days per week for 20 minutes; "insufficiently active" was defined as active at less-than-recommended levels; and "inactive" was defined as no physical activity.

Strength training

Strength training programs should be affordable and accessible and should address issues such as physical limitations and fear of injury. Strength training programs for older adults should be performed 2 or more days per week, and can be performed with no weights, hand and ankle weights, or resistance bands. Exercise should start with no weights and then progress, starting with 1- to 2-lb weights increased slowly as tolerated. Exercises should involve the major muscle groups of the arms, legs, shoulders, chest, abdomen, back, and hips. Two sets of 8 to 15 repetitions of each exercise should be completed with a rest period between sets. The person should not hold his or her breath and should not lock joints in the arms and legs. There should be adequate stretching before and after exercise. Exercises should be stopped any time pain occurs. These recommendations are summarized in Box 3 [16].

Endurance exercises

Endurance exercises should start gradually at as little as 5 minutes at a time, especially if there has been a long period of inactivity. Time should increase to a goal of 30 minutes on most or all days of the week. Initially this time can be divided into 10-minute sessions.

Endurance exercises include any activity that raises heart rate and breathing for an extended period of time. These include activities such as walking, jogging, and swimming.

Balance exercises

Balance exercises can be performed using a stable chair and can be practiced with the patient in the office. Some basic exercises include plantar flexion (toe raises standing behind the chair), knee flexion (extending/flexing the knee standing behind a chair), and hip flexion (raising the leg, flexing at

---

Box 3. Strength training recommendations for older adults

- Exercises should be performed 2 or more days per week.
- Certain exercises can be performed either standing or seated.
- Use hand and ankle weights, resistance bands, or no weights at all.
- If weights are used, start with 1 to 2 lb and gradually increase the weight over time.
- Perform exercises that involve the major muscle groups (eg, arms, shoulders, chest, abdomen, back, hips, legs) and exercises that enhance grip strength.
- Perform 8 to 15 repetitions of each exercise, then perform a second set.
- Do not hold breath during strength exercises.
- Rest between sets.
- Avoid locking joints in arms and legs.
- Stretch after completing all exercises.
- If at any time pain is felt, stop exercising.

Data from Centers for Disease Control and Prevention. Strength training among adults aged ≥ 65 Years—United States, 2001. MMWR Morb Mortal Wkly Rep 2004;53(2):25–8.

the hip standing behind a chair). Two others are hip extension (bending forward over a chair and lifting the leg backward) and the side leg raise (abducting the leg while standing behind a chair).

Strength exercises

A simple upper extremity strength exercise is the arm raise (sitting in an armless chair with feet flat on the floor and arms straight down at the sides, then raising the arms up to shoulder level, holding for 1 second, repeating 8 to 15 times, and eventually adding weights). Another exercise that can be added after the patient has been doing the arm raise for a month or so is the biceps curl in which the patient sits in an armless chair, holding the hands to the side with weights. The patient then slowly bends one elbow up toward chest, holds for 1 second, then repeats with the other arm and alternates for 8 to 15 repetitions. For lower extremity strengthening, it is recommended that the patient do plantar flexion (8 to 15 toe raises standing behind a chair, followed by rest and repeat). To increase quadriceps strength, knee extension exercises can be recommended. The patient should sit in a stable chair, raise leg in front as straight as possible, hold 1 to 2 seconds, and do 8 to 15 repetitions for each leg. Rest and then repeat.

Stretching exercises

Stretching exercises should be performed before and after strength and endurance exercises, three to five times at each session. The stretch should be held for 10 to 30 seconds. If the patient has had a hip replacement, the legs should not be crossed unless clearance is obtained from an orthopedic surgeon. The patient should not stretch to the point of pain or bounce the stretch at the end of the stretching range. Possible stretching exercises include the hamstrings stretch (sit sideways on a bench keeping one leg stretched on the bench with the toes up and the other leg off the bench; straighten the back and hold the stretch for 10 to 30 seconds until the stretch is felt; repeat three to five times on each side) and the Achilles stretch (stand with hands against the wall, arms outstretched, knees bent; step back 1 to 2 feet with heel and foot flat on the floor until the stretch is felt; hold 10 to 30 seconds; repeat three to five times for each side). Another is the wrist stretch in which the hands are placed together in the praying position, the elbows are raised so that the arms are parallel to the floor, the position is held for 10 to 30 seconds, and then the action repeated three to five times. The quadriceps stretch requires the person to be on a firm bed or the floor and on the side so that the hips are aligned one above the other. The head is rested on an arm or pillow while the top knee is flexed so that the ankle can be grasped and gently pulled back until the thigh stretches. The stretch if held for 10 to 30 seconds and then repeated three to five times.

Resources

An excellent reference available free of charge in hard copy and on the Internet is provided by the National Institute on Aging, titled "Exercise: A Guide from the National Institute on Aging." The guide includes step-by-step instructions on exercises in endurance, strength, balance, and stretching, with animated illustrations, charts, and other resource contacts [17]. It is available at http://niapublications.org/exercisebook/toc.htm. The free exercise guide can be ordered along with a video or printed off the Internet. It is also available in Spanish.

Also recommended are "Anytime, Anywhere" exercises to improve balance (eg, walk heel to toe, stand on one foot, stand up and sit down on a chair without using hands) [17]. Tai Chi exercises have also shown to improve balance.

Additional information on strength training in older adults can be found at: http://www.cdc.gov/nccdphp/dnpa/physical/growing_stronger/growing_stronger.pdf. A Tool Kit to Prevent Senior Falls can be found at http://www.cdc.gov/ncipc/pub-res/toolkit/toolkit.htm. And the American Geriatrics Society has a patient education form, "A Patient's Guide to Preventing Falls," available on the Internet at http://www.healthinaging.org/public_education/pef/falls_and_balance_problems.php.

Achieving lifestyle change

Continuation of exercise over time is important, but maintaining motivation can be a problem that is difficult for a person of any age to overcome. Having someone in the family or community in addition to the primary care provider to encourage continuation of the exercise and resistance training can be of great assistance. Organized programs that include the exercises outlined above and found on the suggested Web sites can be developed at senior centers, health clubs, hospitals, churches, or any other organizations that cater to older persons. Participating in a regular exercise program is a major lifestyle change for some people, and it is probably unrealistic to think that they will do this independently. The current cohort of older adults has looked forward to retirement to enjoy "the good life." For most, this concept has led to a sedentary lifestyle with gradual decline in physical activity. The office-based practitioner is in a position to reverse this view.

Assistive devices

Assistive devices can be helpful for patients who have a history of falls caused by factors such as muscle weakness associated with conditions such as a stroke, or structural compromise associated with arthritis. Walkers offer stability and may be of benefit for patients who have arthritis. Walkers provide sideways stability but do not prevent backward falls. A cane, which provides minimal stability, should be used on the side opposite a weak or painful limb. Proper cane length is determined by holding the cane with the elbow in 20° to 30° of flexion to provide optimal support [13]. Patients who have a history of falls or increased fall risk should be considered for hip protectors. Some studies have shown up to a 60% reduction in the risk for hip fractures when hip protectors are worn, especially in nursing home populations. The hip protectors must be worn 24 hours a day. One report has questioned the effectiveness of hip protectors [18], but for now they should be recommended for patients who are at high risk for falling and who will wear them. Other interventions to consider in reducing the risk for fall injury are to place the bed lower to the floor or to use a padded mat next to the bed. Finally, treating osteoporosis is an important interventional strategy. In general, all older women and many older men should receive 1200 to 1500 mg of calcium and 400 to 800 IU of vitamin D each day in addition to recommendations to avoid tobacco, to participate in weight-bearing exercise, and to avoid more than moderate alcohol consumption. Bisphosphonates should be prescribed for women who have T scores below −2 on bone mineral density testing in the absence of risk factors and below −1.5 if risk factors are present.

Summary

Determining fall risk can be a daunting task for the busy clinician, but a simple set of questions and observations at each encounter with the patient can help. Rarely does a complete fall-risk evaluation have to be completed in one visit. Most patients will have a gradual or incremental decline and the evaluation can be performed over time.

The clinician should ask the older patient at each visit if he or she has had a fall, is concerned about falling, or is concerned about balance or gait. The clinician should also take notice of the person's mobility at the time of each encounter and observe how the patient enters the office and the examination room. How did the person get on the examination table room? Did the person walk in independently or with the aid of a family member or office staff? By being vigilant in the evaluation of patients at each visit, the office practitioner can more easily identify subtle declines that may lead to disability, falls, and the potential injuries associated with falls. Once at-risk patients are identified, risk factors can be reduced or eliminated and ongoing exercise and fitness programs recommended.

Acknowledgments

The authors would like to thank Michelle M. Kost, Research & Evaluation Assistant, and Ulric R. Fuller, Coordinator, Michigan State University, Department of Family & Community Medicine, Division of Research, for their assistance in the literature search. This Research

Division is funded by a U.S. Department of Health and Human Services–Health Resources and Services Administration Academic Administrative Units in Primary Care grant (2D54HP00101-04-00).

References

[1] Falls and Fall Risk Clinical Practice Guideline 1998. American Medical Directors Association. Available at: http://www.amda.com. Accessed February 21, 2005.

[2] AGS Panel on Falls Prevention. Guideline for the prevention of falls in older persons. J Am Geriatr Soc 2001;49(5):664–72.

[3] Vyrostek SB, Annest JL, Ryan GW. Surveillance for fatal and nonfatal injuries–United States, 2001. MMWR Surveill Summ 2004;53(7):1–57.

[4] Federal Interagency Forum on Aging Related Statistics. Older Americans 2004: Key Indicators of Well-Being (Older Americans 2004). Washington, DC: U.S. Government Printing Office; 2004.

[5] Rubenstein LZ, Josephson KR. The epidemiology of falls and syncope. Clin Geriatr Med 2002;18(2):141–58.

[6] Cali CM, Kiel DP. An epidemiologic study of fall-related fractures among institutionalized older people. J Am Geriatr Soc 1995;43(12):1336–40.

[7] Tinetti ME. Performance-oriented assessment of mobility problems in elderly patients. J Am Geriatr Soc 1986;34(2):119–26.

[8] Tinetti ME, Doucette J, Claus E, et al. Risk factors for serious injury during falls by older persons in the community. J Am Geriatr Soc 1995;43(11):1214–21.

[9] Leipzig RM, Cumming RG, Tinetti ME. Drugs and falls in older people: a systematic review and meta-analysis: I. psychotropic drugs. J Am Geriatr Soc 1999;47:30–9.

[10] Leipzig RM, Cumming RG, Tinetti ME. Drugs and falls in older people: a systematic review and meta-analysis: II. Cardiac and analgesic drugs. J Am Geriatr Soc 1999;47:40–50.

[11] Tinetti ME, Speechley M, Ginter SF. Risk factors for falls among elderly persons living in the community. N Engl J Med 1988;319(26):1701–7.

[12] Alexander N. Falls. In: Beers MH, editor. Merck manual of geriatrics. 3rd edition. Whitehouse Station (NJ); Merck & Co.: 2000. p. 195–203.

[13] Rubenstein LZ, Solomon DH, Roth CP, et al. Detection and management of falls and instability in vulnerable elders by community physicians. J Am Geriatr Soc 2004;52:1527–31.

[14] Lipsitz LA. Hypotension. In: Beers MH, editor. Merck manual of geriatrics. 3rd edition. Whitehouse Station (NJ); Merck & Co.: 2000. p. 847.

[15] Podsiadlo D, Richardson S. The timed "Up and Go": a test of basic functional mobility for frail elderly persons. J Am Geriatr Soc 1991;39(2):142–8.

[16] Centers for Disease Control and Prevention. Strength training among adults aged $\geq$ 65 Years—United States, 2001. MMWR Morb Mortal Wkly Rep 2004;53(2):25–8.

[17] National Institute on Aging. Exercise: a guide from the National Institute on Aging. Available at: http://niapublications.org/exercisebook/toc.htm. Accessed February 21, 2005.

[18] van Schoor NM, Smit JH, Twisk JWR, et al. Prevention of hip fractures by external hip protectors. JAMA 2003;289(15):1957–62.

ELSEVIER
SAUNDERS

Prim Care Clin Office Pract
32 (2005) 699–722

PRIMARY CARE:
CLINICS IN
OFFICE PRACTICE

Urinary Incontinence: Basic Evaluation and Management in the Primary Care Office

Linda J. Keilman, MSN, APRN, BC[a,b,*]

[a]College of Nursing, Michigan State University,
516 Tarleton, East Lansing, MI 48824, USA
[b]Geriatric Education Center of Michigan, Michigan State University,
B215 West Fee Hall, East Lansing, MI 48824, USA

Urinary incontinence (UI) is the involuntary loss of urine in any amount, from a few drops to total emptying of the bladder. Although UI has received much media and pharmaceutical attention in the last 2 decades, some clinicians still do not ask about urine leakage or offer evaluation and intervention. In addition, patients and health care providers may consider UI a normal part of aging. Although the prevalence of UI increases with age, the condition is not normal or inevitable. Furthermore, with appropriate evaluation and targeted interventions, UI and its associated symptoms can be relieved and the consequences mitigated. This article presents a basic overview of UI in the older adult and an approach to its evaluation and management in the primary care office–based setting. UI in other settings, such as the nursing home and hospital, and UI in younger adults is not addressed.

Scope of the problem

UI occurs in 14% to 25% of community-dwelling older individuals [1]. Prevalence increases with age, with one third of women over age 65 years experiencing some degree of UI and 12% reporting daily urine leakage [2]. In men, prevalence ranges from 3% to 11% [3]. Thirty percent to 40% of individuals over age 75 years will develop urinary urgency and frequency, often with associated leakage [4]. Faced with so prevalent a condition, office-based clinicians should periodically ask each older adult in the practice about UI and initiate a simple, systematic evaluation when it is present.

---

* 516 Tarleton, East Lansing, MI 48823.
  E-mail address: keilman@msu.edu

0095-4543/05/$ - see front matter © 2005 Elsevier Inc. All rights reserved.
doi:10.1016/j.pop.2005.06.003

Estimated direct and indirect costs related to UI are staggering, with estimates at $28 billion or more annually [5]. Direct costs include provider visits, diagnostic studies, and medical and surgical interventions, whereas indirect costs include personal expenses for laundering, dry cleaning, absorbent products, specialty undergarments, and specialty barrier and skin cleansing products. Annual expenditures to manage UI rival those of many chronic diseases in women especially, with expenditures for women over age 65 years reported to be twice that for women under age 65 years [6].

These monetary costs notwithstanding, the most profound cost of UI may be on quality of life. Although most clinicians working with older adults recognize that maintaining function and independence is important, the connection between UI, function, and quality of life may not always be obvious. Active older adults who develop UI or who experience worsening UI symptoms often give up community activities (eg, volunteering, church attendance), hobbies (eg, bird watching, hiking), lifelong interests (eg, theater, musical events), and traveling. Older adult women with UI also report a decreased desire to be sexually intimate because of urine leakage. This insidious withdrawal from these important life events and experiences may eventually lead to social isolation, low self-esteem, spiritual distress, hopelessness, depression, functional decline, and falls and fractures. Research findings even suggest a relationship between UI and mortality, especially in older frail men [7], and UI has long been considered a risk factor for nursing home placement [8,9]. A more recent report, however, suggests that UI may not be an independent risk factor for death, nursing home admission, or functional decline [10]. Therefore, it is important to determine how UI affects each individual in terms of functional status and quality of life. One of the available quality-of-life tools can be used to measure the impact that UI has on an individual's life experience and feelings of well-being [11].

Nighttime UI with or without frequency or urgency can also have an adverse effect on function and quality of life. Although the number of arousals for urination increases with age, it should not interfere with the sleep experience. Generally, one or two trips to the bathroom during the night are considered usual with aging. Most individuals are able to fall back to sleep easily. Problems may arise when individuals get up three or more times at night and have difficulty returning to restful sleep. This decreased amount of sleeping time can lead to daytime drowsiness and even confusion in some patients, which may interfere with the performance of activities of daily living or instrumental activities of daily living [11].

Age-related changes

Age-related changes usually occur gradually and progressively. A number of age-related changes in (and outside) the urinary system may predispose the older adult to the development of urinary incontinence [12]. Specific age-related changes can be magnified in the presence of comorbidities, certain medications, and lifestyle choices. A brief overview of the physiologic and age-related changes that may contribute to UI is presented in Table 1 [11,13,14].

Evaluation

Perhaps the most important aspect of evaluating and managing UI in the office setting is for the clinician to initiate dialog by asking the question, "Do you ever leak urine or have difficulty getting to the toilet in time?"

Table 1
Some age-related changes that may contribute to urinary incontinence

Changes	Impact
Decrease in bladder elasticity and capacity	Increased frequency in voiding
Decrease strength of detrusor muscle	Incomplete emptying of the bladder
Spontaneous detrusor muscle contractions or increased muscle hyperactivity	Urge symptoms
Detrusor muscle laxity	Large, atonic bladder leading to insufficient intravesicular pressure to initiate urination [13]
Mass and renal weight decreased	Decreased surface area available for filtration
Decreased renal blood flow	Drugs excreted through the kidney require dose adjustment
Kidneys less efficient at concentrating urine	Increase in urine volume
Enlargement of the prostrate gland	Decreased flow, difficulty initiating the urine stream, hesitancy, voiding prolonged
Decreased estrogen production	Changes perineum health
Female external urinary sphincter atrophies	Relaxation of the pelvic floor
Diurnal and nocturnal production of urine altered related to circadian sleep-awake pattern	Nocturia episodes increased; increased risk for falls
Changes in antidiuretic, atrial natriuretic and renin aldosterone hormones [14]	Nocturia
Atrophic vaginitis and urethritis	Decreased urethral mucosal seal, irritation, more prone to urinary tract infections
Decreased overall bone mass; spinal column curved and compressed; degenerative changes in joints	Decreased hand dexterity leading to inability to manipulate belts, suspenders, zippers and buttons on clothing; increased pain on ambulation; slower movement
Decreased muscle mass and strength	Falls or fear of falling [11]
Decreased pupil size, visual acuity, ability to accommodate	Decreased ability to adjust to changes in lighting, poor eyesight [11]

Partly due to the persistence of aging myths, women in particular believe that urine leakage is part of growing older. Generally, these individuals will not bring up the topic voluntarily. In addition to the myth that UI is a normal part of aging, other reasons for not broaching the subject may include embarrassment, fear of getting older and facing one's own mortality, fear of surgery, fear of taking another medication, expense, and the belief that there is no effective treatment. It has been estimated that fewer than 50% of individuals experiencing urine leakage report the problem to their health care provider [15,16]. Even when patients bring up symptoms of UI, only 40% receive information about treatment options [17]. After UI is recognized, an evaluation should follow. A caveat is that the amount and frequency of the incontinence should not be the determining factor in proceeding with an evaluation. If it is of concern to the patient, then evaluation is warranted.

The purpose of a systematic evaluation of UI is fourfold: (1) to identify reversible or transient causes of UI and individual patient risk factors, (2) to determine the actual or potential effect of UI on the patient's quality of life and functional status, (3) to anticipate and address potential complications based on established causes [13], and (4) to develop a set of interventions that targets the risk factors and causes for each patient through a consistent approach to evaluation.

According to the updated 1996 UI guideline developed by the Agency for Health Care Policy and Research (now the Agency for Health Care Research and Quality), the goals of evaluation are to confirm the presence of UI, to identify all current conditions that may be contributing to UI, to identify patients who require further evaluation, and if possible, to arrive at a diagnosis [18]. The guideline also emphasizes the concepts of preventing UI symptoms and promoting healthy bladder habits [19]. Both of these concepts confirm the importance being able to recognize each patient's risk factors, including current and past lifestyle choices.

Transient UI usually refers to leakage or other symptoms of relatively new onset and is often based on factors outside the urinary system. Transient UI may be temporary or reversible. Up to one third of community-dwelling older adults with UI may have transient UI [20]. Determining and treating the underlying cause or causes generally lead to resolution of the incontinence [21]. The clinician can use the mnemonic "DIAPPERS" to recall the causes of transient UI [11,22,23]. Although this mnemonic is useful in triggering the clinician's memory, it can also be viewed as disrespectful. One should not associate aging and UI with diaper products. Undergarments for older adults with UI should be referred to as absorbent products, briefs, or other neutral terminology to help eliminate the image that old people with incontinence are just like babies. The causes of transient UI are listed in Box 1 [14,24]. As stated earlier, successful management of the underlying cause or causes may often eradicate the incontinence.

Box 1. Causes of transient or reversible urinary incontinence

D—Delirium; dementia; other confusional states

I—Infections: urinary (symptomatic), respiratory, skin

A—Atrophic vaginitis, urethritis; alcohol ingestion; acute illness

P—Psychologic causes: depression, grief/loss, spiritual distress, hopelessness

P—Pharmacologic agents (including side effects): diuretics, sedative/hypnotics, anticholinergics, α-adrenergic blockers, α-adrenergic agonists, calcium channel blockers, antidepressants, antipsychotics, narcotic analgesics, antiparkinsonism medications, some angiotensin-converting enzyme inhibitors [14,24]

E—Endocrine disorders (hypercalcemia, hyperglycemia); excess urine output; excessive fluid intake; pedal edema

R—Restricted mobility: physical restraints, musculoskeletal disorders, inappropriate or no assistive devices, environmental barriers, lack of caregiver assistance

S—Stool impaction; chronic constipation; fecal incontinence

If UI persists after addressing any potential transient causes or if no transient causes are identified, then the next step in the process is to identify risk factors. Many older adults may have more than one risk factor for UI. The more risk factors an individual has, the more likely she or he will develop UI. The more risk factors that can be successfully addressed, the better the chances for decreasing the incontinence and associated symptoms. The most common risk factors are listed in Box 2 [9,11,13,25–43]. The clinician and patient should work together to identify and address as many of these risk factors as possible.

History

The clinician should obtain a focused history about UI, followed by a detailed review of the medical and surgical history to identify pre-existing or comorbid conditions. A systems review can identify sensory or mobility problems and cognitive or emotional disorders [44] and elicit clues to a change in functional status, weight, eating habits, or fluid intake [45].

During the focused history, patients should be questioned about usual bladder habits; frequency; urgency; leakage with coughing, sneezing, laughing, bending, or lifting; difficulty starting and maintaining the urine stream; postvoid dribbling; a feeling of bladder fullness that persists after urination; and straining to complete the voiding process [46]. Clinicians should ask about urinary tract infections and urinary tract procedures,

Box 2. Risk factors associated with urinary incontinence

Increasing age [25,26]
White race [26,27]
Sex: female-to-male ratio (2:1) over age 60 years [28]
Higher level of education [29]
Perimenopausal status related to decreased estrogen [30]
Increased body mass index [30]
Increased caffeine intake [31]
Impaired functional status [27]
Decreased cognition, delirium [13]
Medications: diuretics, psychotropics, narcotics, anticholinergics,
    α-adrenergic agonists and antagonists, cholinergic agonists
    [32,33]
Medication noncompliance (eg, not taking prescribed diuretic
    for heart failure related to wanting to "avoid accidents") [9]
Ingestion of food or beverages known to be bladder irritants:
    carbonated beverages, milk/milk products, citrus juices and
    fruits, highly spiced foods, tomatoes and tomato products,
    sugar, honey, corn syrup, artificial sweeteners, caffeine (coffee,
    tea, cola, chocolate) [34]
Current smoker or history of smoking [30,35]
Alcohol consumption [36]
Chronic constipation, fecal impaction, fecal incontinence [11,26]
Pregnancy-related factors: mode of delivery, increased parity,
    fetal birth weight [28,37,38]
History of abdominal, gynecologic, rectal, or prostate surgery;
    pelvic radiation [25,39]
Benign prostatic hyperplasia [36]
Presence of comorbid conditions, particularly diabetes,
    hypertension, arthritis, congestive heart failure, Parkinson's
    disease, chronic obstructive pulmonary disease
    [26,30,34,36,40]
Impaired mobility [11,41,42]
Decreased hand dexterity [43]
Pain: chronic, acute, undertreated [9]
History of stroke [26,36]
Depression [9,13]
Environmental barriers [43]
Lack of caregiver assistance [13]
Athletic lifestyles or high-impact physical activity in younger
    years [38]

including catheterization. Nighttime voiding habits, sleep and rest patterns, usual activity pattern, bowel habits, dysuria, and pain on urination also are important aspects of the history-gathering process. Duration and severity of all symptoms should be assessed [47]. Asking the patient about prior interventions and outcomes may also be informative.

If possible, the clinician should ask the patient to complete a 24-hour dietary recall or a similar instrument to collect information about usual dietary habits, favorite foods and drink, and alcohol consumption. Reviewing the form with the patient may provide a better understanding about eating and drinking patterns and consumption of potential of bladder irritants. In addition, because many older adults engage in socialization at mealtime or at other food- or drink-related activities, this is a logical place to ask about social support and relationships.

Questions about living arrangements and the environment should also be posed. Lighting, steps, rugs and floor covering, location and number of bathrooms, and distance required to get to the bathroom may be important on a case-by-case basis. For example, an older community-dwelling adult may have a bathroom on the second floor yet spend the daytime hours on the first level of the home. Under these circumstances, it may be easy to understand why urine leakage occurs while ascending the stairs to get to the bathroom. Such information allows the clinician to make positive suggestions that may enable the person to maintain independence with relatively modest changes (eg, in this case, keeping a urinal or portable commode in a private area on the first floor).

A urinary symptom/voiding diary (Table 2) or bladder log can pro-vide patient-reported information that may be beneficial to the clinician. Some experts in UI consider the voiding diary to be one of the most important components of the evaluation [48] and suggest that it be sent to the patient along with instructions before the office visit to evaluate incontinence. Then, at the time of the office visit, the diary can be the focal point of the encounter and serve as the framework for collecting the historical information, as described earlier. When reviewing the diary, the clinician looks for patterns and associations. How frequent are the symptoms and is there any regularity? What activity was occurring at the time of leakage? Does consumption of a particular food or beverage seem to be associated with urge, incontinence, or both? In the author's experience, even frail older adults living independently are capable of keeping an accurate diary for 3 days. The sample diary shown in Table 2 is too small for many older adults to read and fill out, so it should be configured with a larger font and more room to jot notes in the boxes. This is best accomplished by placing the diary double-sided on a sheet of paper. The sample diary in Table 2 has an area at the bottom for the patient to record the number of pads used and a space to record the number of times that under garments or clothes needed to be changed. A section for bowel movements can also be helpful in diagnosing constipation. Finally, the diary

Table 2
Urinary symptom/voiding diary

URINARY SYMPTOM/VOIDING DIARY   NAME: DATE: DAY#: _____

TIME	FOOD		DRINK		ACTIVITY/FEELING	TOILET	LEAKAGE
	WHAT?	AMOUNT?	WHAT?	AMOUNT?		AMOUNT	AMOUNT
Sample	Wheat toast/dry	2 slices	OJ	6 oz glass (1)	Washing dishes	X small	
5–6 AM							
6–7 AM							
7–8 AM							
8–9 AM							
9–10 AM							
10–11 AM							
11–noon							
12–1 PM							
1–2 PM							
2–3 PM							
3–4 PM							
4–5 PM							
5–6 PM							
6–7 PM							
7–8 PM							
8–9 PM							
9–10 PM							
10–11 PM							
11–12 mid							
12–1 AM							
1–2 AM							
2–3 AM							
3–4 AM							
4–5 AM							

Number of Pads Used: _____   Number of Times Clothes or Undergarments Changed: _____

can be used as a monitoring tool to determine the effectiveness of interventions.

Older adults often are on numerous medications, and a thorough review should be accomplished at least yearly. Asking patients to bring in all of the medications they have at home is a common approach used to gain perspective on past and current health issues. This technique has been called the "brown bag test" by some investigators [49]. It is important to review not only prescription medications but also all nonprescription drugs, home remedies, supplemental/herbal therapies, and caffeine and alcohol intake. Many times, in doing a medication review, the clinician discovers the potential reason for the patient's UI. Any suspicious medication should be decreased or carefully discontinued if possible. If the patient requires a particular class of drugs, substituting another drug in the same class with a different side-effect profile can be considered [24].

Physical examination

The physical examination helps the clinician clarify possible causes of transient UI, detect underlying conditions and causes associated with persistent UI, evaluate comorbid conditions, and determine functional ability [48]. General appearance, skin integrity, and cardiopulmonary status are important indicators of overall patient health. In addition, the clinician should look for lower extremity edema, palpate peripheral pulses, and check for venous insufficiency.

Functional status, especially mobility, is considered one of the keys for controlling UI [11]. Mobility status should be assessed, in part, when the older adult is not aware of the observation. A good time to do this is when staff escort the patient to the examination room. Is there an assistive device? If so, is it being used appropriately? Does the patient hold on to the wall or others for support in the absence of assistive devices? Does the patient require a rest period? The clinician should consider the gait pattern and balance. What type of shoe is the patient wearing? Is this his or her usual footwear? In the examination room, how does the patient get on and off the examination table or up and down from the chair? When the clinician enters the examination room, the hand should be extended to the patient for a handshake, which can provide information about vision, strength, dexterity, and gross coordination—all integral aspects of the toileting experience and manipulation of clothing.

From a practical perspective, the neurologic examination should include a measure of cognition. Does the person have sufficient cognition to recognize the stimulus to urinate, to find the bathroom, and to perform sequential toileting tasks? Lower extremity and perineal sensation, dexterity, strength and balance, and anal and bulbocavernosus reflexes should be assessed [4,21]. On abdominal examination, the clinician should look for diastasis recti, masses, hernias, ascites, and organomegaly that can influence intra-abdominal pressure and urinary tract function [50]. Is there tenderness in the suprapubic region or evidence of bladder distention?

Part of the examination should be performed with a full bladder if the patient is able to tolerate it. To accomplish this, the patient can drink water during the history portion of the visit or come to the appointment with a full bladder. A full bladder allows the clinician to perform the evoked cough response or stress test and to conduct prevoid bladder scanning if the office has access to a portable bladder scanning device. Stress testing, when performed accurately, has a sensitivity and specificity of greater than 90% [48]. The maneuver is performed in two positions to determine the degree of pelvic organ support. First, the patient is positioned comfortably in a supine position, knees bent, and feet resting on the examination table. The abdominal assessment can be performed first and then the perineum can be examined. The clinician should step to the side of the examination table, visualize the urethral meatus, and ask the patient to cough [51]. The test is positive if there is any leakage of urine. The clinician should estimate the amount of leakage and the timing in relationship to the cough. The prevoid bladder scan can be completed next. The patient is assisted off the examination table, asked to stand upright with legs slightly spread and knees bent, and instructed to cough again. Leakage that starts with the cough is considered a positive finding. False negatives are possible for a variety of reasons, including presence of a large cystocele, less-than-full bladder, or patient inability to relax the pelvic floor. Following the tests for stress incontinence, the patient should provide a clean-catch midstream urine specimen and empty the bladder. After the patient has emptied the bladder, the bladder can be scanned or an in-and-out catheterization can be done to determine postvoid residual volume, which is discussed further later.

The gynecologic examination in some older women may need to be approached in a conservative manner, keeping it as minimally invasive as possible [52]. The clinician should assess for perineal dermatitis and look for signs of atrophy, prolapse, vaginal stenosis, or scar tissue [24,44]. The clinician may want to forego using a speculum and perform a digital vaginal examination instead [52].

In examining men, the glans penis should be examined for evidence of circumcision or mobility of the foreskin [24]. The clinician should assess testicular symmetry, tenderness, or enlargement. The prostate is palpated for nodularity, tenderness, and size. Enlargement of the prostate does not necessarily correlate with urethral obstruction but should raise suspicion and consideration for further evaluation [44].

For men and women, the rectal examination should include looking for skin irritation, perianal lesions, and symmetry of the gluteal creases and checking for fecal impaction, the presence of stool in the anal canal, masses, hemorrhoids, sphincter tone, and perianal sensation. The same sacral roots (S2-4) innervate the external urethral sphincter and the anal sphincter [48]. If stool is present, it should be tested for occult blood. The ability of the older patient to tolerate this portion of the examination should always be considered. Providing explanations about what is being done and why can make the examination tolerable for the patient, allowing the clinician to gain valuable information.

Diagnostic studies

The diagnostic tests conducted for patients with UI not only help to clarify the diagnosis but also help to direct treatment decisions and to inform prognosis [53]. As described in "History," prevoid, portable, non-invasive ultrasonography (scanning the bladder) should be performed with the patient's bladder full. This test provides an estimate of bladder capacity. The postvoid residual volume is an essential component of the UI evaluation and should be performed within 5 minutes of an intentional void [54]. When determining postvoid residual volume, bladder scanning is preferable to in-and-out catheterization because of the potential for trauma and infection, but not all primary care clinics have access to bladder scanners. A postvoid residual volume of 50 mL or less is considered normal. A postvoid residual volume of 50 to 100 mL is suggestive of weakness or possible obstruction. A postvoid residual volume greater than 100 mL is considered abnormal and a residual volume greater than 200 mL may indicate the need for referral [2].

Urinalysis by dipstick testing is useful in eliminating bladder infection and in detecting the presence of glucose, protein, and hemoglobin [26]. If dipstick findings are negative, then the specimen does not need to be sent for laboratory evaluation. If the sample is positive, it should be sent for microscopy, culture, and sensitivity. Further diagnostic tests should be ordered only if the results would change treatment interventions [55].

Classification of urinary incontinence

Identification of UI, with or without a definitive diagnosis, is a priority [56]. After UI is identified, continued evaluation in the primary care office or by a consultant should provide information about its underlying cause and allow it to be classified into one of the standard categories: stress, urge, mixed stress/urge, overflow, and functional (Table 3).

A history of urine leakage during periods of increased abdominal pressure (laughing, sneezing, lifting) suggests a diagnosis of stress UI [54]. Feelings of urge or the inability to prevent urine leakage before arriving at the bathroom is generally considered urge UI. Urge UI occurs most commonly in older women [47]. The diagnoses of stress, urge, and mixed UI can usually be determined during the history [2]. A history of continual dampness or frequent dribbling may indicate a diagnosis of overflow UI [54]. There are not clear-cut symptoms that identify UI as functional, but after other types of incontinence are ruled out, functional UI becomes

Table 3
Interventions for urinary incontinence

Type of UI	Intervention	Reference
Stress: leakage that occurs with increased abdominal pressure (coughing, laughing, sneezing, bending, lifting, stepping); inadequate urinary sphincter function; pelvic floor musculature laxity	Patient education	[2,13,14,18,26,28,42, 45,52,54,61,67]
	Pelvic floor muscle exercise or Kegel exercise	
	"Timed voiding"—toileting on a fixed schedule that is consistent; 2 h while awake is typical; also referred to as Scheduled Voiding	
	"Habit training"—utilizing the toilet at a set time interval based on findings from voiding diary; generally starting 30 min before leakage occurs; intervals can be adjusted related to the individual's voiding pattern; goal is to gradually increase the intervals between voiding without leakage	
	Diet modification (related to bladder irritants)	
	Avoid caffeine and alcohol intake	
	Weighted vaginal cones	
	Pessaries and other intravaginal devices (requires manipulation, manual dexterity, and scheduled monitoring by the provider)	
	External occlusive device (for men and women)	
	Intraurethral occlusive device (urethral plug for women, requires manipulation and manual dexterity)	
	Pelvic floor electrical stimulation	
	Preventive skin care	
	External collection device (condom catheter with leg bag for men)	
	Absorbent products	
	Medication review	
	Biofeedback	
	Collagen injections	
	Surgery	

Urge: sudden overwhelming need to urinate without ability to control initiation of urine flow, whether bladder is full or not; uncontrolled detrusor contractions or detrusor hyperactivity

Patient education
Pelvic floor muscle exercise
Timed voiding
Habit training
"Urge inhibition"—resisting or inhibiting the urge to urinate; stopping current activity, relaxation, and distraction techniques including thinking about something other than urinating; counting backward from 100 by 7; "quick flicks," or squeezing and releasing pelvic floor muscle quickly; delay urge for only 10–20 min, and then continue to the bathroom
"Bladder training"—starting with a short voiding interval (usually every hour) and gradually increasing (usually 2- to 3-h intervals) time between toileting, with the goal of staying dry and suppressing the urge
Diet modification
Fluid management
Avoid caffeine and alcohol intake
Voiding diary for 2–3 wk with detailed information
Preventive skin care
Absorbent products
External collection device
Medication review
Anticholinergic agent
Temporary, intermittent catheterization (requires manipulation and dexterity)

[2,13,14,18,51,52,67]

(continued on next page)

Table 3 (*continued*)

Type of UI	Intervention	Reference
Mixed: combination of urge and stress symptoms	Directed at whichever type of UI seems to be predominant Patient education Pelvic floor muscle exercises Timed voiding Habit training Bladder training Urge inhibition Diet modification Fluid management Avoid caffeine and alcohol intake Preventive skin care Absorbent products Medication review Electrical stimulation	[2,52,67]
Overflow: involuntary leakage of urine in small amounts that is frequent or constant; associated with incomplete bladder emptying and reduction in the force of the urine stream	Patient education "Double-voiding technique"—attempting to void twice during one trip to the bathroom; patient may void, sit for 2–10 min, then try revoiding; if stable, may stand up, press abdomen up toward chin, sit down, then try revoiding "Cred'e maneuver"—using one or both hands to press firmly on the abdomen over the bladder during voiding to facilitate emptying Diet modification Avoid caffeine and alcohol intake Preventive skin care External collection device Absorbent products Use of barrier product to prevent skin breakdown Medication review Surgery	[4,14,18,67,68]

[14,17,18,67]

Functional: recognition of the urge to urinate but unable to physically get to the toilet, unable to ask for assistance, or no motivation to toilet; related to cognitive and functional status; diagnosis of exclusion

Patient education

Appropriate assistive mobility devices in close proximity at all times

Environment alterations to allow easier access to toilet (increase lighting, remove clutter)

Use of elderly-friendly furniture for ease of maneuverability (arms on chairs, firm cushion seats)

Adjustment to toilet facility (raised seat, grab bars)

Consider adaptable clothing (elastic, snaps, Velcro)

Preventive skin care

Caregiver assistance

Caregiver education

"Prompted voiding"—setting an alarm clock or kitchen timer to remind older adults living alone to utilize the toilet facility; caregiver reminds or asks the patient to utilize the toilet on a regular schedule, generally every 2 h during waking hours; also called "routine toileting"

Absorbent products

Check for possible underlying depression or cognitive impairment and treat the condition

Alternative toiletry device use (urinal, bedpan, bedside commode)

Consider referral to physical or occupational therapy

Medication review

Use of substitute toiletry devices (urinal, bedpan, bedside commode), especially at night

For poor vision: regular eye examinations, current eyeglass prescription, glasses available at all times (consider neck chain), remove old prescriptive lenses from home (can donate)

(continued on next page)

Table 3 (*continued*)

Type of UI	Intervention	Reference
Nocturia: wakes during the night one or more times to urinate	Patient education No fluid 2 h prior to bedtime (fluid restriction) Decrease caffeine and alcohol intake Medication adjustment for diuretics to be taken no earlier than mid afternoon to early evening Voiding diary for 1–2 wk Padding the bed/mattress instead of wearing tight briefs overnight	[11,20,51,54]
Other		
Constipation, fecal impaction	Removal of impaction Nutritional consult to determine appropriate fluid and fiber intake Bran/applesauce/prune juice recipe Appropriate stool softeners Accurate bowel record Maintain at least three stools a week that are soft, formed, and evacuated without straining	[11,13]

a presumptive diagnosis, given the patient's cognitive and functional status and self-report of specific difficulties [57].

Treatment and management interventions

Every older adult's life experience is unique, as is each person's experience with UI. Effective treatment requires a multifaceted approach that focuses on the level of individual patient understanding and the impact of UI on quality of life and function. The first choice for treatment should be the least invasive treatment that has the least number of potential complications. The clinician should keep in mind that the least invasive treatment may not lead to the best outcome in certain situations [48].

Behavior modification other behavioral therapies, lifestyle changes, and environmental interventions are first-line treatments for UI, with the goals of improved quality of life, maintaining function, and enhancing self-esteem. The clinician does not need the definitive UI diagnosis to begin treatment of UI with behavioral therapies and lifestyle changes [53]. Any clinician should be able to use behavioral modification as part of the UI management plan. Interventions are simple, relatively inexpensive, effective, and do not have significant adverse effects [45]. In one research study, patients who received a behavioral management intervention at home decreased UI severity by 61% compared with the control group whose UI severity increased by 184% without behavioral management [58]. Table 3 lists some common interventions for the common types of UI. All behavioral interventions require active participation and motivation on the part of the patient with UI; therefore, these interventions may not be suitable for some individuals with depression or cognitive impairment or other confusional states [18,59]. All interventions should be individualized and mutually agreed on with the older adult.

The initial step in the management of UI is to correct any transient or reversible causes (see Box 1) [60]. In addition, risk factors (see Box 2) such as obesity, smoking, inadequate fluid intake, and alcohol consumption should be addressed when appropriate. Education is a crucial component in the management of UI [60]. Patients should understand basic urinary system anatomy and physiology and the basic mechanism of micturition. Education helps to dispel myths and can help with compliance. Effective and appropriate health communication materials can be obtained from a number of health care agencies and organizations (Table 4). Office staff can provide patients with appropriate materials or such information can be displayed in the waiting room.

Pelvic floor muscle exercises, or Kegel exercises, provide the foundation for an effective UI management program. Although many women tell the clinician that they are familiar with the exercise, they explain it as being practiced while urinating on the toilet, starting and stopping the urine flow. This method actually disrupts voiding patterns and can lead to retention

Table 4
Resource List UI Materials

Organization	Material	Web address
American Academy of Family Physicians	Patient education	http://familydoctor.org/798.xml?printxml
American Foundation for Urologic Diseases	Patient brochure	http://www.incontinence.org/publications/INCONT.PDF
American Geriatrics Society (AGS)	Patient education brochure	http://www.americangeriatrics.org/products/ui/ui_brochurev2.pdf
Health Care Professional Resource List on UI	Organizations & agencies providing professional & public information	http://www.americangeriatrics.org/products/ui/resource_list.htm
National Institute on Aging	Age Page	http://www.niapublications.org/engagepages/Urinary_Incontinence.pdf
The Merck Institute of Aging & Health	Urinary Incontinence Toolkit: Professional tools & educational material	http://www.miahonline.org/tools/UI/tools.html

and urinary tract infection. The correct method to perform the exercises must be explained to the patient and instructions should be given in writing. It is often helpful to have the patient do several exercises while in the office to confirm that they are being done correctly.

An effective approach to teaching pelvic floor muscle exercises is to ask the patient to imagine trying to "hold back" passing gas (flatus). The patient usually indicates that he or she would "squeeze my butt cheeks together." The clinician can then ask the patient to concentrate on the rectum and imagine pulling or lifting it up through the body to the chin. Patients need to be told not to lift their buttocks, tighten the abdomen or thigh muscles, move their legs, strain down, or hold their breath. In the beginning, the activity should be held for a slow count of 5 to 10 depending on the functional status and frailty of the older adult. The patient is then told to relax for twice as long, or a count of 10 (20 if initially held for 10), to be sure the muscle has returned to baseline and there are no fasciculations. Pelvic floor muscle exercises should be performed in a series of 3 to 5 repetitions at least three times a day while lying, standing, and sitting. Patients should be instructed to do the exercises every day, indefinitely. To begin, the older adult should associate performing pelvic floor muscle exercises while engaged in a daily activity such as mealtime, grooming, or taking medication. This helps promote compliance to the treatment regimen. A minimum of 30 to 45 pelvic floor muscle exercises every day is recommended [4]. It is important to inform the patient that it generally takes from 4 to 8 weeks to see a difference in severity of urine leakage. Pelvic floor muscle exercises have been reported to provide an 81% reduction in urine leakage episodes [61]. It is important to emphasize the need for persistence with these exercises that should become a part of the older adult's normal daily routine. If the exercises are stopped, then the positive benefits gained from performing pelvic floor muscle exercises will be lost because the muscles will atrophy [36].

A variety of devices is available for stress UI, especially for women. The foam pessary, bladder-neck support prosthesis, urethral occlusive devices, and intraurethral devices are just a few. Numerous research studies, however, report poor compliance with many of these devices [28]. The clinician must keep in mind the patient's manual dexterity, visual acuity, and willingness to touch themselves and insert the devices. Decisions on whether to use any of these devices should be individualized and made with the patient. If the patient is not going to use the device, why include it in the treatment plan?

There is a plethora of absorbent products on the market. The clinician should be knowledgeable about what is available and what is appropriate for each patient. Although the expected outcome is to decrease urine leakage, it may still be necessary for the older adult to wear some type of disposable product to allow them to comfortably engage in social activities and decrease the potential smell of urine, thus maintaining or improving their quality of life. The type of pads or protective garments should be individualized based on gender, UI diagnosis, volume of incontinence, and cost [54,55]. The use of products should not foster independence or take away from other desirable treatment [62]. Older adults should be discouraged from using plastic-lined, tight-fitting products during the night because of the potential for skin breakdown and infection related to the warm and moist environment created by various products and urine.

Medications

A number of drugs have been and will continue to be introduced into the UI market. Comparisons between available drug treatments are limited and not much help to the health care provider [2]. It is important to keep in mind that most traditional anticholinergic therapies are limited in their effectiveness [63]. For the treatment of stress UI, anticholinergics are inappropriate and ineffective [2]. Medications for urge incontinence should not be used until other treatment interventions and modalities have failed over a sufficient length of time [64]. Drugs are a major cause of urinary incontinence and urinary retention in the elderly. Many frequently pre-scribed medications can cause urinary symptoms including frequency and urge (see Box 1). Keep in mind that when a patient is receiving a sedative, hypnotic, or analgesic, "any drug that dulls the brain, dulls the bladder, because your brain tells you when you have to void" [51].

Pharmacotherapy may be useful to augment behavioral and lifestyle treatment and management interventions [20]. Drugs can be particularly helpful for women who have prominent urge symptoms, no cardiac problems or cognitive deficits, and can tolerate and address the side effects of dry mouth, blurry vision, or constipation. If possible, the clinician should delete or decrease dosages of current medications that may be contributing to UI before adding a drug to treat UI [11]. The well-known mantra for geriatric pharmacology, "start low and go slow," should be invoked when prescribing a drug for the treatment of UI.

At times, the patient is so distraught about UI that he or she is unable to engage in behavioral interventions at the outset of the treatment process. Prescribing appropriate drug therapy may help the individual gain some control over symptoms and then become more motivated to work on behavioral or lifestyle interventions.

In the future, the treatment of UI may involve pharmacogenomic approaches or even gene therapy [63]. For now, behavioral therapies, lifestyle changes, and environmental enhancement are the interventions of choice. Table 3 lists some of the interventions for specific types of UI.

Referral

UI can be handled effectively in the primary care setting most of the time. Interventions described earlier in this article can be appropriately implemented and monitored by knowledgeable office-based primary care providers. Circumstances for which referral should be considered include:

- Failure to respond to treatment over time
- Increasing symptoms
- Appearance of new symptoms
- Microscopic hematuria in the absence of infection
- Existence of anatomic abnormalities or severe prolapse
- History of prior urologic corrective surgery followed by urine leakage
- Inability to determine a diagnosis after working with the patient for a reasonable length of time
- Positive neurologic findings in the absence of a current diagnosis
- Postvoid residual volume of 200 mL or greater, repeated twice [54,55]

Maintaining positive relationships with health care providers and specialists in the community who have expertise in UI is imperative.

Continence surgery is indicated when conservative treatment fails or the patient wants definitive treatment [26]. Surgery is the final management option for UI [11]. Palliative measures can be used for those patients whose UI is not curable [11].

Summary

With the increasing number of older adults in the population, the office-based clinician can expect to see more people with UI. Continued UI research is warranted, especially research that includes older adults who reside in the community and frail elderly women who are still living in the community [52]. Better outcome measures should be developed to assess the effectiveness of interventions for UI [65]. Reliance on information obtained from voiding dairies is used extensively, yet the reliability and validity for any specific instrument have not been tested with older adults. Hopelessness and spiritual distress, as precursors to health decline and how they impact on quality of life, should be studied in older adults with UI. Given the prevalence of UI, should it be considered a public health problem for which population-based interventions are used [66]?

What is known is that older adults demonstrate significant improvement in symptoms of UI when education, counseling, support, and encouragement in behavior management and lifestyle interventions are provided. When motivated and positive, even frail older adults experience improvement in the severity of urine leakage. Perhaps the single most important action that the office-based clinician can take is to start asking every older adult about UI and to follow with the basic approaches to evaluation and management described in this article.

References

[1] Morley JE. Urinary incontinence and the community-dwelling elder: a practical approach to diagnosis and management for the primary care geriatrician. Clin Geriatr Med 2004;20(3):427–35.

[2] Weiss BD. Selecting medications for the treatment of urinary incontinence. Am Fam Physician 2005;71(2):315–22.

[3] Nitti VW. The prevalence of urinary incontinence. Rev Urol 2001;3(Suppl 1):S2–6.

[4] Newman DK. Managing and treating urinary incontinence. Baltimore (MD): Health Professions Press; 2002.

[5] Wagner TH, Hu TW. Economic costs of urinary incontinence in 1995. J Urol 1998;51(3):355–61.

[6] Wilson L, Brown JS, Shin GP, et al. Annual direct cost of urinary incontinence. Obstet Gynecol 2001;98:398–406.

[7] Johnson TM, Bernard SL, Kincade JE, et al. Urinary incontinence and risk of death among community-living elderly people: results from the national survey on self-care and aging. J Aging Health 2000;12(1):25–46.

[8] Ouslander JG. Urinary incontinence in the nursing home. J Am Geriatr Soc 1990;38:289–91.

[9] Prochoda KP. Medical director's review of urinary incontinence in long-term care. J Am Med Dir Assoc 2002;3(Suppl 1):S11–5.

[10] Holyrud-Leduc JM, Mehta KM, Covinsky KE. Urinary incontinence and its association with death, nursing home admission and functional decline. J Am Geriatr Soc 2004;52(5):712–8.

[11] DuBeau CE. The continuum of urinary incontinence in an aging population. Geriatrics 2002;57(Suppl 1):S12–7.

[12] Elbadawi A, Diokno A, Millard R. The aging bladder: morphology and urodynamics. World J Urol 1998;16(Suppl 1):S10–34.

[13] Bhagwath G. Urinary incontinence in the elderly: pathogenesis and management. Indian Acad Clin Med 2001;2(4):270–5.

[14] Merkelj I. Urinary incontinence in the elderly. South Med J 2001;94(10):952–7.

[15] Weiss BD. Diagnostic evaluation of urinary incontinence in geriatric patients. Am Fam Physician 1998;57(11):2675–90.

[16] Cobbs EL, Ralapati AN. Health of older women. Med Clin N Am 1998;82(1):127–44.

[17] DuBeau CE. The continuum of urinary incontinence in an aging population. Urology Times 2002. Available at: http://www.urologytimes.com/urologytimes/article/articleDetail. jsp?id=20870. Accessed March 1, 2005.

[18] Fantl JA, Newman DK, Colling J, et al. Urinary incontinence in adults: acute and chronic management. Clinical Practice Guideline no. 2, 1996 update. Rockville (MD): US Department of Health and Human Services, Public Health Service, Agency for Health Care Policy and Research; 1996. AHCPR publication 96–0682.

[19] Newman DK. What's new: the AHCPR guideline update on urinary incontinence. Ostomy Wound Manage 1996;42(10):46–56.

[20] Shah D, Badlani G. Treatment of overactive bladder and incontinence in the elderly. Rev Urol 2002;4(Suppl 4):S38–43.

[21] Gibbons L, Choe JM. Helping women quell urinary incontinence. Clin Advisor 2004;7(5): 21–8.

[22] Resnick NM, Yalla SV. Management of urinary incontinence in the elderly. N Engl J Med 1985;313:800–8.

[23] Lekan-Rutledge J, Colling J. Urinary incontinence in the frail elderly. Am J Nurs 2003; 103(Suppl):36–46.

[24] Voytas J. The role of geriatricians and family practitioners in the treatment of overactive bladder and incontinence. Rev Urol 2002;4(Suppl 4):S44–9.

[25] Gray ML. Gender, race and culture in research on urinary incontinence. Am J Nurs 2003; 103(3):S20–5.

[26] Thakar R, Addison R, Sultan A. Management of urinary incontinence in the older female patient. Clin Geriatr 2005;13(1):44–54.

[27] Fultz NH, Herzog AR, Raghunathan TE, et al. Prevalence and severity of urinary incontinence in older African American and Caucasian women. J Gerontol A Biol Sci Med Sci 1999;54:M299–303.

[28] Sampselle CM. Behavioral interventions in young and middle-age women. Am J Nurs 2003; 103(3):S9–19.

[29] Ruff CC, van Rijswijk L, Okoli A. The impact of urinary incontinence in African American women. Ostomy Wound Manage 2002;48(12):52–8.

[30] Sampselle CM, Harlow SD, Skurnick J, et al. Urinary incontinence predictors and life impact in ethnically diverse perimenopausal women. Obstet Gynecol 2002;100:1230–8.

[31] Arya LA, Myers DL, Jackson ND. Dietary caffeine intake and the risk for detrusor instability: a case-control study. Obstet Gynecol 2000;96:85–9.

[32] Ouslander JG. Geriatric considerations in the diagnosis and management of overactive bladder. J Urol 2002;60:50–5.

[33] Johnson T, Ouslander J. Urinary incontinence in the older man. Med Clin N Am 1999;83(5): 1247–66.

[34] DuBeau CI, Bent AE, Dmochowski RR, et al. Addressing the unmet needs of geriatric patients with overactive bladder: challenges and controversies. Clin Geriatr 2003;11(12): 16–27.

[35] Luber KM. The definition, prevalence, and risk factors for stress urinary incontinence. Rev Urol 2004;6(Suppl 3):S3–9.

[36] Josephson KL, Ginsberg DA. Key considerations when treating the older patient with symptoms of urinary frequency and urgency. Ann Long Term Care Clin Care Aging 2004; 12(11):25–32.

[37] Holyroyd-Leduc JM, Straus SE. Management of urinary incontinence in women. JAMA 2004;291(8):986–95.

[38] Nygaard IE, Thompson FL, Svengalis SL, et al. Urinary incontinence in elite nulliparous athletes. Obstet Gynecol 1994;84(2):183–7.

[39] Umlauf MG, Sherman SM. Symptoms of urinary incontinence among older community-dwelling men. J Wound Ostomy Continence Nurs 1996;23(6):314–21.

[40] Brown JS. Epidemiology and changing demographics of overactive bladder: a focus on the postmenopausal woman. Geriatrics 2002;57(Suppl 1):S6–12.

[41] American Medical Directors Association. Urinary incontinence: clinical practice guideline. Columbia (MD): American Medical Directors Association; 1996.

[42] Rosenberg MT, Dmochowski RR. Overactive bladder: evaluation and management in primary care. Cleveland Clin J Med 2005;72(2):149–56.

[43] Ouslander JG. Geriatric considerations in the diagnosis and management of overactive bladder. Urology 2002;60(Suppl 5A):49–55.

[44] Smith DA. Evaluation of urinary incontinence. J Am Med Dir Assoc 2002;3(Suppl 1):S2–10.

[45] Rovner ES, Wein AJ. The treatment of overactive bladder in the geriatric patient. Clin Geriatr 2002;10(1):20–35.

[46] Ouslander JG, Schnelle JF. Incontinence in the nursing home. Ann Intern Med 1995;122(6): 438–49.

[47] Mutone M, Valaitis SR. Practical evaluation of the incontinent woman. Female Patient 2004;29(4):38–44.

[48] Beers MH, Berkow R, editors. Merck manual of geriatrics. 17th edition. Indianapolis (IN): John Wiley & Sons; 1999.

[49] Freml JM, Farris KB, Fang B, et al. Iowa priority's brown bag medication reviews: a comparison of pharmacy students and pharmacists. Am J Pharm Educ 2004;68(2):1–7.

[50] Culligan PJ, Heit M. Urinary incontinence in women: evaluation and management. Am Fam Physician 2000;62(11):2433–52.

[51] Newman DK, Harms D. Addressing the unmet needs of patients with overactive bladder. CE-Today Nurse Pract 2004;3(5):7–16.

[52] Lekan-Rutledge D. Urinary incontinence strategies for frail elderly women. Urol Nurs 2004; 24(4):281–302.

[53] Johnson T. Nonpharmacological treatments for urinary incontinence in long-term care residents. J Am Med Dir Assoc 2002;3(Suppl 1):S25–30.

[54] Imam KA. The role of the primary care physician in the management of bladder dysfunction. Rev Urol 2004;6(Suppl 1):S38–44.

[55] Ouslander JG, Dutcher JA. Overactive bladder: assessment and nonpharmacological interventions. Consult Pharm 2003;18(Suppl B):13–20.

[56] Vogel SL. Urinary incontinence in the elderly. Ochsner J 2001;3(4):214–8.

[57] Jirovec MM. Functional incontinence. In: Urinary and fecal incontinence: nursing management. 2nd edition. St. Louis (MO): Mosby; 2000. p. 145–58.

[58] Dougherty MC, Dwyer JW, Pendergast JF, et al. A randomized trial of behavioral management for continence with older rural women. Res Nurs Health 2002;25(1):3–13.

[59] Schnelle JF, Smith RL. Quality indicators for the management of urinary incontinence in vulnerable community-dwelling elders. Ann Intern Med 2001;135(8):752–8.

[60] O'Hara S, Borrie MJ. Management of urinary incontinence in older women. Geriatr Aging 2004;7(4):35–9.

[61] Burgio KL, Locher LJ, Goode PS, et al. Behavioral versus drug treatment for urge urinary incontinence in older women: a randomized controlled trial. JAMA 1998;280(23): 1995–2000.

[62] Lekan-Rutledge D, Doughty D, Moore KN, et al. Promoting social continence: products and devices in the management of urinary incontinence. Urol Nurs 2003;23(6):416–58.

[63] Chancellor MB. New frontiers in the treatment of overactive bladder and incontinence. Rev Urol 2002;4(Suppl 4):S50–6.

[64] Dmochowski R. Interventions for detrusor overactivity: the case for multimodal therapy. Rev Urol 2002;4(Suppl 4):S19–27.

[65] Engberg S, Kincade J, Thompson D. Future directions for incontinence research with frail elders. Nurs Res 2004;53(Suppl):S22–9.

[66] Sampselle CM, Palmer MH, Boyington AR, et al. Prevention of urinary incontinence in adults: population-based strategies. Nurs Res 2004;53(Suppl):S61–7.

[67] Wyman JF. Treatment of urinary incontinence in men and older women: the evidence shows the efficacy of a variety of techniques. Am J Nurs 2003;(Suppl 3):S26–35.

[68] Dowling-Castronovo A, Bradway C. Urinary incontinence. In: Mezey M, Fulmer T, Abraham I, et al, editors. Geriatric nursing protocols for best practice. 2nd edition. New York: Springer Publishing Co. Inc.; 2003. p. 83–98.

ELSEVIER
SAUNDERS

Prim Care Clin Office Pract
32 (2005) 723–753

PRIMARY CARE:
CLINICS IN
OFFICE PRACTICE

Hypertension in the Elderly

Michael Maddens, MD, CMD[a,b,*],
Khaled Imam, MD, CMD[a], Ayham Ashkar, MD[a]

[a]*Division of Geriatric Medicine, William Beaumont Hospital,
3535 West 13 Mile Road, Suite 108, Royal Oak, MI 48073, USA*
[b]*Wayne State University School of Medicine, Detroit, MI 48201, USA*

From 2001 to 2002, among those 65 years of age and over, 47% of men and 52% of women reported having hypertension. The National Health and Nutrition Examination Survey (NHANES) suggests that among 65- to 74-year-olds, 60.9% of men and 74% of women are hypertensive. Among those 75 years and older, the numbers are 69.2% for men and 83.4% for women [1]. Together with the impending demographic wave (over the next 45 years, the "over 65" population in the United States will double and the "over 85" population will nearly quadruple) [2], high blood pressure (BP) will represent a major challenge to health care providers in this country. Hypertension is more prevalent in elderly women than elderly men and more prevalent in blacks compared with whites (Table 1), with data from the Center for Health Statistics indicating that between 1979 and 1997, death rates related to hypertension rose in elderly white women and in blacks of both sexes [3,4].

Prevalence in the Elderly

The Seventh Report of the Joint National Committee on Prevention, Detection, Evaluation, and Treatment of High Blood Pressure (JNC 7) classification of BPs is outlined in Table 2 [5].

Among older adults with hypertension, isolated systolic hypertension (elevated systolic BP [SBP] with normal diastolic BP [DBP]) predominates over diastolic or combined systolic/diastolic hypertension (Table 3).

* Corresponding author. Division of Geriatric Medicine, William Beaumont Hospital, 3535 West 13 Mile Road, Suite 108, Royal Oak, MI 48073.
  E-mail address: mmaddens@beaumont.edu (M. Maddens).

0095-4543/05/$ - see front matter © 2005 Elsevier Inc. All rights reserved.
doi:10.1016/j.pop.2005.06.002
primarycare.theclinics.com

Table 1
Prevalence of high blood pressure by sex and race among persons over 70 years of age

Group	BP $\geq 140/90$ (%)
Black women	82.9
Black men	67.1
White women	66.2
White men	59.2

Data from Burt VL, Whelton P, Roccella EJ, et al. Prevalence of hypertension in the US adult population: results from the Third National Health and Nutrition Examination Survey, 1988–1991; and Hypertension 1995;25:305–30.

Even when those who have clinical cardiovascular disease or who take antihypertensive agents are excluded, hypertension is more likely to be isolated systolic hypertension, especially in women. By age 80 years, the prevalence of isolated diastolic hypertension is less than 4% [6], and in elderly nursing home residents, isolated diastolic hypertension is even more uncommon (<1%) [7]. Sagie and colleagues [8] reported that among untreated hypertensive patients aged 60 years and older, 76% of men with what is now classified as stage I isolated systolic hypertension will progress to stage II or higher, as will 47% of men whose SBP is less than 140 mm Hg at baseline. Among women, the numbers are 80% and 59%, respectively [8].

In contrast, findings from the Helsinki Aging Study suggest that although SBP increases with age in cross-sectional data, analysis of longitudinal data suggests that BP declines in most individuals at all entry ages (65, 75, 80, and 85 years), with 85-year-old men the only group to have less than half of the individuals experience a drop over the subsequent 5 years. Baseline BP was the single greatest predictor of subsequent decline (explaining 27%–37% of the variance). Baseline BP, age, health status after 5 years, a drop in cholesterol, and a drop in triglycerides were significant predictors of subsequent decline in BP readings [9].

Despite the well-established impact of high BP on health outcomes, a substantial segment of hypertensive patients remains unaware, untreated,

Table 2
Classification of blood pressures

BP classification	Systolic BP (mm Hg)		Diastolic BP (mm Hg)
Normal	<120	And	<80
Prehypertension	120–139	Or	80–89
Stage 1 hypertension	140–159	Or	90–99
Stage 2 hypertension	≥ 160	Or	≥ 100

JNC 7 classification.

Data from Chobanian AV, Bakris GL, Balck HR, et al. The Seventh Report of the The Joint National Committee on Prevention, Detection, Evaluation, and Treatment of High Blood Pressure. JAMA 2003;289:2561.

Table 3
Prevalence of systolic, diastolic, and combined high blood pressure

Group	Isolated systolic	Isolated diastolic	Systolic + diastolic
Men	58%	12%	30%
Women	65%	7%	28%

Adapted from Wiling SVB, Belanger A, Kannel WB, et al. Determinants of isolated systolic hypertension. JAMA 1998;260:3452.

or uncontrolled, with older Mexican American women being the least likely to achieve BP control (Table 4) [10]. Although data from 1999 suggest that over 97% of elderly report having had their BP checked and increasing numbers report having hypertension [11], awareness, knowledge, and attitudes about high BP may be barriers to effective therapy. A nationally representative sample of 1503 adults over age 50 years revealed that only 55% recognized that hypertension and high BP were the same. Only 30% identified hypertension as a serious health concern. Although most had had their BP measured, only 54% knew their BP [12].

Among elderly patients who have uncontrolled hypertension, 80% have isolated systolic hypertension and an additional 14% meet systolic and diastolic criteria [13]. Among elderly persons from the NHANES-III who

Table 4
Awareness, treatment, and control of high blood pressure

Group	% Aware	% Treated	% Controlled
Non-Hispanic blacks			
Men			
50–69 y	73	56	22
70+ y	67	58	25
Women			
50–69 y	84	71	29
70+ y	79	70	23
Non-Hispanic whites			
Men			
50–69 y	71	55	25
70+ y	56	46	16
Women			
50–69 y	81	66	34
70+ y	68	58	19
Mexican Americans			
Men			
50–69 y	54	37	15
70+ y	55	40	12
Women			
50–69 y	70	47	16
70+ y	49	31	7

Data from Burt VL, Whelton P, Roccella EJ, et al. Prevalence of hypertension in the US adult population: results from the Third National Health and Nutrition Examination Survey, 1988–1991. Hypertension 1995;25:305–13.

were unaware of their high BP, 91% had isolated systolic hypertension. The elderly were nearly 8 times as likely to be unaware of their hypertension and nearly twice as likely not to have achieved control even after they were aware [14]. Among elderly nursing home residents with a mean age of 83 ± 8 years, hypertension is listed as a diagnosis on the federally required Minimum Data Set in 32% of patients. Prevalence was higher among women (33%) than men (27%), and among African Americans (43%) and other minorities (34%) compared with whites (30%). With advancing age, the prevalence decreased: 35% in 65- to 74-year-olds, 33% in 75- to 84-year-olds, and 30% in those 85 and older, although most of this difference was accounted for by a decline in the percentage in African American men because prevalence was not affected by age in women. Many patients had comorbidities: 26% had coronary artery disease, 22% had congestive heart failure, and 29% had cerebrovascular disease [15].

Dietary, medication, and environmental factors

Dietary sodium intake is a well-established risk factor for the development of hypertension, whereas increased dietary calcium has been shown in the NHANES-III cohort to be associated with a blunting of the age-related increases in SBP and pulse pressure [16,17]. Potassium intake is associated with lower SBP and DBP, whereas alcohol intake is associated with only lower DBP. In addition, the age-related changes in SBP are attenuated by higher protein intake. Magnesium is not associated with any changes in BP [17].

Gurwitz and colleagues [18] reported that elderly patients on nonsteroidal anti-inflammatory drugs (NSAIDs) are at increased risk for subsequent hypertension. In looking at Medicaid enrollees 65 years old and older in New Jersey, these investigators found that the odds ratio for subsequent initiation of antihypertensive therapy was 1.66 (95% confidence interval [CI]: 1.54–1.80) and was NSAID-dose related. Similar trends were reported by Johnson and coworkers [19] in a meta-analysis not limited to the elderly. Pooled data from randomized placebo-controlled trials revealed that NSAIDs elevated mean BP by 5 mm Hg (95% CI: 1.2–8.7), with no statistically significant difference in the elevation according to antihypertensive drug class or NSAID type (although there was a trend toward greater elevations in patients on β-blockers or vasodilators compared with those on diuretics). In somewhat younger patients (mean age, 50 years), Coates and colleagues [20] reported that pseudoephedrine, found in over-the-counter cold remedies and often listed as an agent that may exacerbate high BP, had no effect on BP or pulse rate when administered at a dose of 60 mg four times a day. Given that elderly patients have a tendency toward blunted α-adrenergic responsiveness [21], it is unlikely that pseudoephedrine in the usual clinical dose has a meaningful effect on the BP of most elderly hypertensive patients. Pseudoephedrine and similar drugs, however, may precipitate urinary retention in elderly men who have prostatic hypertrophy.

Lead exposure has also been shown to be a risk factor for hypertension in postmenopausal women, although not specifically in the elderly [22]. Data from the Framingham Heart Study suggest that in women, obesity in midlife may predict the subsequent development of isolated systolic hypertension [23].

Findings of the Baltimore Longitudinal Study on Aging support an association between an attenuation of the age-related increase in SBP and hormone replacement therapy. For women who were age 65 years at entry, 10 years of hormone replacement therapy was associated with a 6.6 mm Hg rise in SBP compared with a 25.6 mm Hg rise in nonusers [24]. Findings from the Women's Health Initiative, however, raise concern about the safety of hormone replacement therapy.

Among obese individuals, the risk for all-cause mortality appears to increase as body mass index increases, especially for those who also have a high sodium intake. There also appears to be an increased risk of fatal stroke in this group [25].

Finally, genetic predisposition and sleep apnea may play a role in the development of hypertension. Strazzullo and colleagues [26] suggested that DD homozygous polymorphism in the angiotensin-converting enzyme (ACE) gene angiotensinogen M235T may be a risk factor for increasing BP in aging persons. Sleep apnea has also been linked to hypertension, although the association appears to be weaker in those over the age of 80 years [27,28].

Age-related physiologic changes impacting blood pressure and blood pressure regulation

Studies of aging have demonstrated steady increases in mean brachial artery pressure beginning in young adulthood and continuing into the eighth decade, although there are differences between populations in the magnitude of the increase. For example, the increase in a rural population was sub-stantially less than that observed in an urban population [29]. Dilatation of the aorta and large arteries, thickening of arterial walls, increased number of collagen fibers in the arterial wall, decreased glycoprotein content of elastic fibrils, increased mineralization ($CaPO_4$) of the elastin, and increased left ventricular posterior wall diastolic thickness are seen with normal aging [29,30]. Functional changes, including increased arterial wall tension, increased peripheral resistance, and an increased arterial stiffness (even in the absence of overt hypertension), manifest as an increased arterial pulse wave velocity [31], which results in the reflected pulse wave returning sooner. In the elderly, the wave reaches back to the thoracic aorta before the left ventricular ejection period has ended, resulting in a summation of the waves, an increase in the SBP, and workload on the left ventricle [32]. Berry and colleagues [33] reported that independent of other known confounders, older women with hypertension have stiffer large arteries, greater central wave reflection, and higher pulse pressures than older hypertensive men, despite higher mean arterial pressure in men. The investigators postulated that this may partly explain the postmenopausal acceleration in the rate of cerebrovascular and cardiac complications.

Aging is associated with declines in carotid baroreceptor function and β-adrenergic receptor–mediated vascular relaxation and chronotropic response but with preserved response to nitroglycerin [34,35].

Effect of hypertension on cardiovascular physiologic changes of aging

Among those with established hypertension, older patients tend to have higher total peripheral resistance, lower cardiac index and left ventricular ejection rate, lower plasma renin activity, lower central and total blood volume, and lower renal blood flow compared with younger hypertensive patients [35–37]. Older patients who have hypertension do not appear to have the normal age-related increase in sympathetic nervous system activity (as reflected by plasma norepinephrine levels), and cardiopulmonary baroreceptor function that is diminished by hypertension is not further diminished in older patients who have hypertension [38]. In contrast, β-adrenergic receptor responsiveness and baroreceptor sensitivity exhibit modest declines beyond that occurring from aging alone [35,39].

Does high blood pressure have adverse effects in elderly persons?

Epidemiologic evidence from the Framingham Heart Study suggests that hypertension is associated with an increased risk of developing cardiovascular disease, with the risk per millimeter-of-mercury rise in SBP increasing with advancing age, at least through age 70 years [40]. Findings from the Cardiovascular Health Study (community-dwelling elderly aged 65 years and older; average age, 72 years) demonstrate an association between SBP and EKG evidence of myocardial infarction, left ventricular mass, and diastolic (but not systolic) cardiac function. Isolated systolic hypertension is also strongly associated with increased intima-media thickness of the carotid artery [6], and reported to be associated with a high risk of carotid bruit [41]. The risk of cardiovascular disease rises proportionally with increasing DBP above 85 mm Hg in older men; however, this trend is reportedly blunted in older women, with increased risk appearing only after DBPs exceed 104 mm Hg [42]. In a meta-analysis of outcome trials in isolated systolic hypertension (SBP > 160 mm Hg and DBP < 95 mm Hg) in patients over age 60 years, Staessen and colleagues [43] reported that although increasing SBP was associated with increased relative hazard rates for total mortality (relative risk [RR] = 1.26 for each 10–mm Hg increase, $P = .0001$)

and stroke (RR = 1.22 for each 10–mm Hg increase, $P = .02$), the relative risk of coronary events (RR = 1.07 for each 10–mm Hg increase, $P = .37$) was not significantly increased. These investigators also observed an inverse relationship between DBP and mortality. Likewise, 10-year follow-up of the Studio sulla Pressione Arteriosa nell'Anziano study in Italy revealed that SBP (but not DBP) is a strong positive, continuous, independent predictor of total mortality and cardiovascular mortality, even in patients older than 75 years [44]. In addition, the Rotterdam Study demonstrated that 1 SD increase in SBP was associated with a 24% increased risk of myocardial infarction, a 59% increased risk of stroke, and a 21% increased risk of all-cause mortality. Increases (1 SD) in DBP had no statistically significant effect on myocardial infarction or all-cause mortality, and had a lesser (27% increase) effect on stroke risk [45]. Furthermore, at least for those in their 60s and 70s, midlife BP appears to impact the risk of stroke from any given level of current BP [46].

Congestive heart failure

High BP is also a known risk factor for the development of congestive heart failure. Framingham Heart Study follow-up at an average of 17 years revealed that a 20–mm Hg increase in SBP produced a 56% increase in the risk of congestive heart failure. Although DBP also predicted subsequent heart failure, it was a much weaker predictor than SBP or pulse pressure. Separate analysis restricted to patients over age 60 years on entry revealed that this relationship was present. Time-dependent systolic pressure, but not time-dependent diastolic pressure, predicted development of heart failure [47].

Progression of atherosclerosis

Progression of carotid and aortic atherosclerosis is also predicted by high BP. In the Rotterdam Study, SBP (but not DBP) was predictive of progression of atherosclerotic carotid plaques, carotid intima-media thickness, aortic atherosclerosis, and lower-extremity atherosclerosis (assessed by decline in the ratio of the SBP at the ankle to the SBP in the arm [ankle/arm BP index]) [48].

Age-related maculopathy

The risk of age-related maculopathy has been shown to increase with increasing SBP. In the Rotterdam study, each 10–mm Hg increase in SBP was associated with an 8% increase in the odds of age-related maculopathy (odds ratio = 1.08, 95% CI: 1.03–1.14) [49].

Effect of high blood pressure on cognition

Hypertension appears to have a negative impact on cognition, although findings are not entirely consistent from study to study. Among young elderly (mean age, 72 years), Kuo and colleagues [50] reported that each 10–mm Hg increase in supine SBP was associated with a 2.31-fold increased risk of impairment in psychomotor speed and set shifting, although there was no impact on tests of verbal fluency, memory, or visuospatial functions. Wallace and coworkers [51] reported that free recall memory was decreased among elderly patients with diastolic (but not systolic) hypertension. Glynn and colleagues [52] found that although current BP was not well correlated with cognitive functioning, BP from 9 years before cognitive testing demonstrated a U-shaped association with the number of errors on memory testing (Short Portable Mental Status Questionnaire). Error rates were 9% higher in patients with SBP less than 130 mm Hg and 7% higher among those with SBPs of 160 mm Hg or greater. Petitti and coworkers [53] reported that retrospective review of charts of patients who had dementia revealed that systolic pressures increased less over time in those who eventually developed dementia, and the diastolic drop that was seen over time in all groups was the most pronounced among those eventually developing dementia. de Leeuw and colleagues [54] reported that duration of hypertension correlated with the volume of periventricular and sub-cortical white matter lesions seen on MRI. The Cardiovascular Determinants of Dementia study reported that among 65- to 75-year-olds, current and previous BP (SBP and DBP) were predictive of severe subcortical and periventricular white matter lesions. In addition, although more rapid increases in systolic pressure over time were predictive of subcortical and periventricular severe white matter changes, these changes were seen with increases and decreases in diastolic pressure compared with prior readings [55]. Sacktor and colleagues [56] compared hypertensive patients by degree of BP control and found that compared with those who had a mean SBP of 135 to 150 mm Hg, those who had an SBP of 135 mm Hg or less had accelerated memory decline (particularly delayed recall), as did those who had an SBP greater than 150 mm Hg (particularly free recall). In the Systolic Hypertenion in the Elderly Program (SHEP) trial, dementia developed in 1.6% of the intervention group versus 1.9% of the placebo group (but one third of the placebo group were on active treatment by year 3) [57].

In the Systolic Hypertenion in Europe (Syst-Eur) trial, Mini-Mental State Exam scores decreased with decreasing diastolic pressures ($P = .04$) in the placebo group but not in the active treatment group. In addition, active treatment of systolic hypertension in this trial was associated with a 50% reduction in the incidence of dementia [58]. Open-label extension of the trial revealed that compared with the controls, long-term antihypertensive therapy reduced the risk of dementia by 55%, from 7.4 to 3.3 cases per 1000 patient years (43 versus 21 cases, $P < .001$). After adjustment for sex, age, education, and entry BP, the relative hazard rate associated with the use of nitrendipine was 0.38 (95% CI: 0.23–0.64, $P < .001$). The data suggest that treatment of 1000 patients for 5 years could prevent 20 cases of dementia (95% CI: 7–33) [59]. Finally, in the Rotterdam Study, antihypertensive therapy resulted in a decreased risk of vascular dementia (adjusted RR 0.3, 95% CI: 0.11–0.99) and an insignificant 13% reduction in Alzheimer's disease [60].

Circadian variation in blood pressure

Blood pressure varies over the course of the day. Among younger nonhypertensive and hypertensive individuals, BP is usually lowest in the early morning hours, peaks in the afternoon, and then begins to decline [61]. Variations in the timing and magnitude of circadian variation have been associated with increased pathology, although findings have not necessarily been consistent. Using ambulatory BP monitoring, Pasqualini and colleagues [62] demonstrated that elderly patients whose nighttime decrease in BP was less than 10% ("nondippers") tended to have poorer quality of sleep and were more likely to be using benzodiazepines. Among 131 asymptomatic elderly patients who had hypertension but not pre-existing cerebrovascular disease, diabetes, or renal insufficiency, Kario and co-workers [63] reported that the prevalence of silent cerebrovascular insults was lowest in patients whose nighttime reduction was between 10% and 20% but was comparably elevated in nondippers (nighttime BP decreased <10%) and in extreme dippers (nighttime BP decreased ≥20%). Left ventricular hypertrophy and microalbuminuria were more prevalent only in nondippers. In contrast, Nakamura and colleagues [64] demonstrated that among patients who already had cerebrovascular disease and who were on antihypertensive therapy, recurrent stroke and the development of new silent ischemic lesions on MRI were (1) more common in those whose nighttime mean arterial BP was at least 10 mm Hg lower than the daytime mean arterial BP compared with individuals on treatment whose day–night difference was less than 10 mm Hg, and (2) comparable to individuals who remained untreated for hypertension.

Patient evaluation

The JNC 7 recommends that physical examination should (1) include at least two measurements of BP with a properly calibrated and validated instrument of appropriate cuff size, (2) be performed with the patient seated with feet on the floor and arm supported at heart level, and (3) use the auscultatory method [5]. The JNC 7 further recommends that SBP be defined as the point at which the first of two or more sounds is heard (phase 1) and DBP as the point before the disappearance of sounds (phase 5), and that the readings and the goal BPs be provided verbally and in writing to the patient. If Korotkoff's sounds disappear and then reappear during cuff deflation, this presence of an auscultatory gap should be noted. An auscultatory gap is more common in the elderly and associated with increased arterial stiffness and an increased prevalence of carotid atherosclerosis [65]. It should be noted that in elderly persons and in those who have isolated systolic hypertension or peripheral atherosclerosis, cuff DBPs are consistently higher than intra-arterial readings by 10 to 18 mm Hg [32,33]. Cuff measurement of SBPs in elderly patients has been reported to underestimate by 4 to 7 mm Hg [34] and insignificantly overestimate intra-arterial readings [33]. When excessive atherosclerosis is present, however, it may require pressure simply to compress the artery, independent of the actual intra-arterial BP, leading to spurious elevations in indirect sphygmomanometric readings (often referred to as pseudohypertension). When pseudohypertension is suspected (eg, with disproportionate symptoms after modest lowering of BP), one should consider performing Osler's maneuver or obtaining BP using an automated device that uses the infrasonic recorder method. Osler's maneuver is performed by assessing the palpability of the pulseless radial or brachial artery distal to the cuff occlusion after the cuff is inflated above systolic pressure. When either of these arteries is palpable with the cuff inflated above systolic pressure, Osler's maneuver is said to be positive. In Osler-positive patients, mercury sphygmomanometry overestimates BP by 10 to 54 mm Hg [35]. The infrasonic recorder may be more accurate in reflecting intra-arterial pressure. Hla and Feussner [66] reported that an infrasonic recorder-cuff difference of 4 mm Hg or greater is sensitive in detecting patients whose cuff reading is greater than 10 mm Hg above their intra-arterial reading. The method is only moderately specific, however, and requires confirmation with direct intra-arterial measurement.

Recording of phases 1, 4, and 5 has been advocated in patients in whom there is a large difference between phase 4 (muffling of Korotkoff's sounds) and phase 5 (disappearance of Korotkoff's sounds), in patients who have hyperthyroidism or aortic insufficiency, and in patients after exercise [67].

Common errors in indirect BP measurement include observer bias, faulty equipment, and failure to standardize the measurement technique [67]. A full review of this subject is beyond the scope of this article. Readers interested in more details about specific measurement issues are referred to (www.nhlbi.nih.gov/health/prof/heart/hbp/bpmeasu.pdf). In the authors' experience, errors commonly encountered in practice include not palpating the brachial artery to ensure that the cuff has been inflated above systolic pressure (rather than into the auscultatory gap), not raising the arm to the level of the heart, and terminal digit preference (most commonly for 0 or 5), which may be avoided by use of an automated device [68]. Practitioners are reminded to calibrate aneroid devices periodically because one study reported that up to 80% of aneroid sphygmomanometers at university hospitals and clinics were found to yield unreliable measurements [69].

In addition, in interpreting BP measurements, clinicians should be aware of the normal decline in pressure that occurs after meals in elderly patients, typically most pronounced within the first hour [70] and more pronounced in hypertensive elderly patients. Postprandial declines of 10 mm Hg or greater are reportedly associated with an increased risk of leukoariosis and lacunar infarction [71], and postprandial readings below 115 mm Hg systolic in frail elderly have been reported to be associated with falls [72].

At the initial visit and on subsequent visits when prompted by symptoms or the addition of medications that increase the likelihood of orthostatic hypotension, measuring BP after the patient is supine for at least 5 minutes and then after standing for 1 to 2 minutes may be useful. Orthostatic hypotension is a risk factor for falls, syncope [73,74], and stroke [75]. Orthostatic declines in diastolic pressure predict cardiovascular mortality [76]. Despite concern over the potential of aggravating the orthostatic changes, cautious treatment of hypertension appears to decrease the likelihood of orthostasis [77].

Although not advocated by the JNC 7 as part of the routine assessment, where available, Doppler BP in all four extremities may be worth consideration at the initial visit. This methodology allows calculation of the ankle/arm BP index, which has been demonstrated to be a sensitive and specific marker of peripheral vascular disease in the elderly, predictive of survival [78], and a predictor of carotid arterial disease among those who have isolated systolic hypertension [79].

As recommended by the JNC 7, initial evaluation of the patient with hypertension should include physical examination, routine laboratory studies, and further diagnostic procedures as indicated after the initial evaluation. Although the utility of most of the individual components of the examination has not been well documented, in addition to an appropriate measurement of BP in both arms, initial physical examination should include height and weight (to calculate body mass index); auscultation for carotid, femoral, and abdominal bruits; and palpation for the presence of an abdominal aortic aneurysm. Funduscopic examination should be performed to determine the presence of hypertensive retinal changes and to assess for the presence of age-related macular degeneration that is more prevalent in elderly hypertensive patients [49]. Palpation of the abdomen should seek to detect enlarged kidneys or masses. Palpation of the thyroid, a thorough examination of the heart and lungs, and a neurologic examination including a baseline cognitive assessment should be performed. Finally, the presence of edema and the status of the peripheral pulses should be noted.

The JNC 7 advises that routine diagnostic studies at initial evaluation should include EKG, serum potassium, creatinine, glucose, calcium, hematocrit, lipid profile, and a urinalysis. In the SHEP trail, participants with baseline EKG abnormalities experienced a greater percentage reduction in subsequent cardiovascular events with treatment than did those with normal EKG at baseline [57]. Assessment of concomitant obesity and hyperlipidemia is advised as noted previously, with the caveat that at advanced age, total cholesterol no longer adds predictive value. In the European Working Party on High Blood Pressure in the Elderly trial, the association of body mass index with outcomes depends on age, treatment status, and the outcome variable of interest, such that no particular ideal body mass index can be comfortably derived from the data. Patients whose body mass indexes were slightly above the population mean of 27 kg/m^2 had the lowest risks [80] and, independent of other risk factors and treatment, mortality in this cohort decreased 14% for each 1-mmol/L increase in pretreatment serum total cholesterol [81]. Additional studies should be guided by results of the initial evaluation or the presence of difficult-to-control BP.

Although not a JNC 7 recommendation, an echocardiogram may be more reliable than an EKG to evaluate left ventricular hypertrophy. In patients who show left ventricular hypertrophy on echocardiogram, consideration should be given to obtaining a urinary albumin/creatinine ratio. This ratio has been shown in diabetic and nondiabetic elderly to predict increasing risk for cardiovascular morbidity and mortality among hypertensive patients who have left ventricular hypertrophy [82].

What is the role for ambulatory blood pressure monitoring in the elderly?

Ambulatory BP monitoring is not routine for elderly patients. Using participants of the Syst-Eur trial, Staessen and colleagues [83] reported that ambulatory BP monitoring in elderly patients with untreated systolic hypertension adds to the ability to predict mortality, cardiac events, and stroke. Nighttime BP (12 AM–6 AM) more accurately predicted end points than daytime level. Untreated patients with a 10% increase in their night/day ratio were 41% more likely to experience an event. Among treated patients, the additional predictive power was lost.

Because all of the major intervention trials for hypertension in the elderly used seated BP as their standard measurement, clinicians using ambulatory monitors should recognize that average 24-hour BP readings correlate less well with casual SBP readings in the elderly (young, $r = 0.69$; elderly, $r = 0.42$) and that casual readings have been reported to run 17 to 28 mm Hg higher than 24-hour average readings with ambulatory monitors [61,83,84]. Clinic–ambulatory differences are higher with advancing age and increasing clinic SBP [84]. For a discussion of technical issues with ambulatory monitors, the reader is referred to www.nhlbi.nih.gov/health/prof/heart/hbp/bpmeasu.pdf.

What is the significance of "labile hypertension"?

Although "labile hypertension" is often believed to have less clinical significance than "fixed hypertension," data from the Framingham Heart Study cohort demonstrated that within-person variation of SBP increases steadily with advancing age. Although labile hypertension is associated with an increased risk of cardiovascular disease, multivariate analysis considering age and baseline BP reveals that lability of pressure is not an independent predictor of cardiovascular risk. Clinicians are advised to not simply accept the lowest of several office BP readings but to calculate the average of the readings [85].

Can the clinician base treatment on self-recorded blood pressure monitoring when the patient has difficulty making it to the office for blood pressure checks?

Although done by many physicians and endorsed by the JNC 7 as potentially benefiting patients by providing information on response to antihypertensive therapy, by improving medication adherence, and in evaluating the possibility of white-coat hypertension [5], the practice benefit of having elderly patients record their own BP at home is unproved. There are little data on the accuracy and predictive value of this practice in the elderly. Although one study in patients with a mean age of 61 years in rural Japan demonstrated that ambulatory SBP readings were more predictive of subsequent mortality than office SBPs [86], another report from that study indicated that isolated systolic hypertension (mean age of subjects, 71.6 years) did not reach statistical significance in predicting cardiovascular disease mortality rate (relative hazard = 1.49, 95% CI: 0.89–2.47, $P = .13$) [87]. Furthermore, Hitzenberger and Magometschnigg [88] reported that self-monitoring is not associated with improvement in the number of patients achieving normotension.

A meta-analysis of studies examining self-reported BPs (largely in younger patients) suggested that a self-recorded SBP of 125 mm Hg was equivalent to a conventional office BP of 140 mm Hg, and a self-recorded DBP of 79 mm Hg corresponded to a conventional reading of 90 mm Hg [89]. Turnbull and colleagues [90], however, reported that patient self-recorded BPs using an automated oscillometric device were 4.7 (SBP) and 2.7 (DBP) mm Hg higher than those recorded by a trained nurse using the automated device or a standard mercury sphygmomanometer. Studies in younger hypertensive patients have demonstrated that left ventricular hypertrophy remains substantially more common in patients whose office BPs are elevated compared with those who are at target BP, despite similarly controlled home BPs [91]. For a discussion of technical issues related to home BP monitoring, the reader is referred to www.nhlbi.nih.gov/health/prof/heart/hbp/bpmeasu.pdf.

Treatment

Thijs [92] observed the increasing effect of placebo on BP reductions with advancing age and noted the necessity for placebo-controlled trials to assess the effect of age on therapeutic responses. There is evidence in the elderly that pharmacologic and nonpharmacologic interventions may be beneficial.

Nonpharmacologic treatment

Several studies have suggested that hypertension in elderly patients is more sensitive to dietary sodium intake [93–96]. Geleijnse and colleagues [97] reported that a sodium:potassium:magnesium (8:6:1) salt substitute used at the table and in food preparation resulted in a 7.6/3.3–mm Hg reduction in BP in the salt substitute group compared with controls who used common table salt, and produced a 28% decrease in urinary sodium excretion. It should be noted that although the elderly are more likely to be salt sensitive, BP may increase in some patients in response to sodium restriction [98]. In addition, a potentially unintended consequence of dietary salt restriction may be decreased iodine intake because in many communities, iodized salt constitutes a major source of iodine intake [99].

Potassium supplementation has inconsistently shown small hypotensive effects; however, there is insufficient evidence in the elderly to make a specific recommendation. Encouragingly, higher intake of potassium is associated with a reduction in stroke-associated mortality, independent of other known cardiovascular risk factors [100,101].

In a small trial, Applegate and colleagues [102] reported that a multifactorial nonpharmacologic intervention (weight reduction, sodium restriction, and exercise) in patients (average age, 65 years) reduced BP by 4.2/4.9 mm Hg compared with controls. In perhaps the largest randomized, controlled trial of nonpharmacologic interventions in the elderly, Whelton and coworkers [103] reported that among subjects 60 to 80 years old whose BP was less than 145/85 mm Hg at entry, sodium restriction (hazard ratio [HR] $= 0.69$, 95% CI: 0.59–0.81, $P < .0010$) and weight loss in obese persons (HR $= 0.70$, 95% CI: 0.57–0.87, $P < .001$) resulted in lower use of BP medication, fewer new diagnoses of hypertension, and fewer cardiovascular events.

Biofeedback has also been explored as a nonpharmacologic option in the elderly, but no outcome trials are available. A small study in elderly patients with isolated systolic hypertension revealed a modest decline in BP. Average monthly professionally measured BP fell significantly, from 164.7/87.1 to 156.9/81.5 mm Hg [104].

Finally, although no intervention data are available specifically in the elderly, smoking has been demonstrated to be associated with an increased risk of coronary heart disease, and the increased risk has been shown to decline to nonsmoker levels within 1 to 5 years after cessation [105].

Pharmacologic treatment

There are several major studies that have focused on elderly patients or included them as a substantial component of the study cohort (Table 5). Choice of initial agent depends on the presence or absence of "compelling indications." For example, the JNC 7 recommends that for patients who have heart failure, diuretics, β-blockers, ACE inhibitors, angiotensin receptor blockers, and aldosterone antogonists are all accepted therapeutic agents. For patients who have sustained a myocardial infarction, β-blockers, ACE inhibitors, and aldosterone antogonists are recommended. For patients who have diabetes, all of these agents except angiotensin receptor blockers are advised. For patients who have chronic kidney disease, ACE inhibitors and angiotensin receptor blockers are recommended. For patients who have had a stroke, diuretics and ACE inhibitors are suggested [5].

A Department of Veterans Affairs Cooperative Study demonstrated that 78% of patients could achieve target BP results with 25 mg of hydro-chlorthiazide, and 89% with 50 mg daily [106]. SHEP reported no difference in the benefit achieved when analyzed by age, race, or sex [107]. In a meta-analysis of outcome trials in isolated systolic hypertension (SBP > 160 mm Hg and DBP < 95 mm Hg) in patients over age 60 years, Staessen and colleagues [43] reported that treatment was associated with a 13% reduction in total mortality (95% CI: 2–22, $P = .02$), an 18% reduction in cardiovascular mortality, a 26% reduction in cardiovascular complications, a 30% reduction in stroke, and a 23% reduction in coronary events. The number needed to treat for 5 years to prevent one major cardiovascular event was lower in patients over age 70 years (19 versus 39), in men (18 versus 38), and in those who had previous cardiovascular complications (16 versus 37). Hemorrhagic and ischemic strokes are reduced with therapy [108]. Beneficial effects have also been variously reported to include reductions in congestive heart failure [109], dementia [58–60], and left ventricular mass. Antihypertensive treatment had a favorable effect on left ventricular mass index (RR = 0.6, 95% CI: 0.4–0.9) regardless of whether treatment used ACE inhibitors, diuretics, β-blockers [110], or calcium channel blockers, with some suggestion that calcium channel blockers may have a greater effect than β-blockers [111].

Applegate and colleagues [112] evaluated the effect of various degrees of SBP control in patients whose "on-treatment" DBPs were less than 90 mm Hg. Compared with patients whose SBPs were at times greater than 160 mm Hg but averaged 151 mm Hg, those whose SBPs were consistently greater than 160 mm Hg (mean, 184 mm Hg) and those whose SBPs were always under 160 mm Hg (mean, 137 mm Hg) had higher cardiovascular morbidity and mortality rates, with rates 50% higher in the "tighter control" group compared with the "moderate-control" group.

Although the Antihypertensive and Lipid-Lowering Treatment to Prevent Heart Attack Trial [113] has suggested the superiority of thiazide diuretics, the Second Australian National Blood Pressure Study suggested that ACE inhibitors may be more beneficial. The latter study included over 6000 patients (51% women) aged 65 to 84 years (mean age, 72 years) who had SBPs of 160 mm Hg or greater or DBPs of 90 mm Hg or greater, with those having SBPs of 140 mm Hg or greater randomized to ACE inhibitors or to diuretics as initial therapy. At 5 years, BP had decreased 26/12 mm Hg in both groups. The outcome (all cardiovascular events and all-cause mortality) rate was lower in patients allotted to the ACE inhibitor group

Table 5
Large trials of high blood pressure in the elderly

Study	Type of HTN	Age (y)	Exclusions	Entry BP (mm Hg)	Target BP (mm Hg)	Drugs	Significant outcomes
SHEP [57] (randomized, blinded, placebo-controlled)	S	60+	Variety of cardiac conditions; insulin; anticoagulants; dementia; Cr >2.0 mg/dL; COPD; EtOH abuse; cancer; life-threatening illness; live in nursing home	S >159 D <90	Lower of S <160 or 20 below baseline	Placebo versus chlorthalidone, then add 1 of: reserpine, metoprolol, hydralazine, or placebo	Stroke; CHF; CV events; CV mortality; dementia
EWPHE [139] (double-blinded, placebo-controlled)	C	60+	Curable causes of HTN; grade II or IV retinopathy; cerebral hemorrhage; hepatitis; cirrhosis; gout; cancer; IDDM	S = 160–239 D = 90–119	S <160 and D <90	HCTZ/triamterene, then add methyldopa	Total CV; total cardiac; MI
Syst-Eur [58,59] (randomized double-blinded)	S	60+	Standing SBP <140; secondary HTN; retinal hemorrhage or papilledema; CHF; dissecting AA; Cr >2 mg/dL; severe epistaxis; MI or CVA within 1 year; dementia, substance abuse; inability to stand; severe CV or non-CV disease	S = 160–219 D <95	S ≥20 below baseline or S <150	Nitrendipine, then add enalapril ± HCTZ	Total stroke; nonfatal stroke; nonfatal cardiac events; total cardiac events; total CV events; dementia

VA Cooperative Trial [106] (randomized, controlled)	D	30–69	Secondary HTN; a variety of medical conditions	D = 95–109	D ≤90	Stepped care versus referral to community care	All-cause mortality (subgroup age 60–69; $P = .08$)
Rotterdam Study [45,48,49,60,110] (prospective population-based cohort)	C	>55	Patients diagnosed with dementia at the time of enrollment	S ≥160 D ≤95	Observation	Not applicable (observation study)	Dementia; chronic disabling cardiovascular, neurologic, locomotor, and ophthalmologic diseases
LIFE [82] [randomized double-blinded parallel group]	E	55–80 with LVH	Secondary HTN; MI or CVA within 6 mo; angina requiring BB or CCB; CHF; EF <40%	S = 160–200 and/or D = 95–115	S ≤140	Losartan vs atenolol	Stroke; New DM (both favored by losartan); cardiovascular death
NORDIL [144] [prospective randomized, open, blinded endpoint]	D	50–74	Patients currently on anti-HTN Tx (unless met entry criteria at 2 visits 1 wk apart off meds]	D ≥100	D <90	Diltiazem, then ACEI, then AB versus diuretic and/or BB, then ACE, then AB	Total stroke (favored by diltiazem regimen)
STOP-II [145,146] (randomized, double-blinded, controlled; 6614 patients)	E	70–84	SBP >230 mm Hg; DBP >120 mm Hg; orthostatic SBP drop >30; MI or CVA in last year; angina requiring meds × NTG; severe/incapacitating illness	S ≥180 and/or D ≥105	<160/95	Conventional (atenolol, metoprolol, or HCTZ + amiloride) versus newer agents (enalapril, lisinopril, felodipine, or isradipine)	No differences in outcomes between "old" and "new" drugs

(continued on next page)

Table 5 (continued)

Study	Type of HTN	Age (y)	Exclusions	Entry BP (mm Hg)	Target BP (mm Hg)	Drugs	Significant outcomes
STOP-1 [147] (randomized, double-blinded, controlled; 1627 patients)	E	70-84	SBP > 230 mm Hg; DBP > 120 mm Hg; SBP ≥ 180 but DBP <90; Orthostatic SBP drop > 30 mm Hg; MI or CVA in the last year; angina requiring meds × NTG; severe/incapacitating illness	180–230/ ≥90 or D: 105–120	S <160/95	Any of: atenolol, HCTZ + amiloride, metoprolol, pindolol, (then add other class if needed)	Stroke + death; total mortality
MRC [148] (randomized placebo-controlled, single-blinded)	B or S	65–74	Secondary HTN; on HTN meds; CHF; Tx for angina; MI or CVA in last 3 mo; renal insufficiency; DM; asthma, K ≤3.4 or >5.0	S: 160–209 and D: <115	S <150 (if entry S <180); S <160 if entry S = 180–209	Atenolol or HCTZ + amiloride or placebo	Stroke; CV events; (both favored by diuretic only)
ANBP-2 [114,149] (randomized [allocation concealed], blinded outcome assessors)	E	65-84	Life-threatening illness; Cr >2.5 mg/dL; malignant HTN; dementia	S: ≥160 or D: >90 (with S ≥140)	Decrease S by 20 or <140, and decrease D by 10 or <90	ACEI or diuretic for initial Tx (at discretion of PMD)	CV events + all-cause mortality (favored ACEI)

Abbreviations: AA, aortic aneurysm; AB, alpha blocker; ACEI, ACE inhibitor; ANBP-2, Second Australian National Blood Pressure Study; B, both systolic and diastolic hypertension; BB, β-blocker; CCB, calcium channel blocker; CHF, congestive heart failure; Cr, creatinine; COPD, chronic obstructive pulmonary disease; CV, cardiovascular; CVA, cerebrovascular accident; D, diastolic; DM, diabetes mellitus; E, either systolic or diastolic hypertension; EF, ejection fraction; EtOH, alcohol; EWPHE, European Working Party on High Blood Pressure in the Elderly; HCTZ, hydrochlorthiazide; HTN, hypertension; IDDM, insulin-dependent diabetes mellitus; K, potassium; LIFE, losartan intervention for endpoint reduction in hypertension study; LVH, left ventricular hypertrophy; meds, medication; MI, myocardial infarction; MRC, Medical Research Council; NORDIL, Nordic Diltiazem study; NTG, nitroglycerin; PMD, primary medical doctor; S, systolic; STOP-I, Swedish Trial in Old Patients with Hypertension I; STOP-II, Swedish Trial in Old Patients with Hypertension II; Tx, treatment; VA, US Department of Veterans Affairs.

compared with the diuretic group (odds ratio = 0.89, 95% CI: 0.79–1.00). The difference in the number needed to treat was 3.7; however, the upper confidence limit of the number needed to treat was greater than 400, suggesting that although the difference was statistically significant, it was not likely clinically significant [114].

Special populations

Are diuretics effective in elderly patients who have mild renal dysfunction?

The SHEP trial investigators evaluated the effect of mild renal dysfunction on the effectiveness of chlorthalidone in treating systolic hypertension. Compared with patients who had normal creatinine, patients who had serum creatinine 1.35 to 2.40 mg/dL achieved similar BP reductions (with no additional deterioration in renal function) and were less likely to develop hypokalemia [115].

What evidence is there for benefit of treatment among elderly hypertensive patients who have diabetes?

Treatment of hypertension using diuretic therapy in younger patients who have diabetes has previously been reported to be associated with excess mortality [116]; however, this does not appear to be a problem in the elderly. Tuomilehto and colleagues [117] conducted a subgroup analysis of the Syst-Eur trial participants to assess the benefits of treating elderly patients who had diabetes and isolated systolic hypertension. They found that patients who had diabetes benefited from treatment and that the magnitude of the benefit was greater in patients who had diabetes compared with those who did not (Table 6).

Table 6
Effect of diabetes on outcomes of treatment of high blood pressure [117]

Outcome	Diabetic patients: adjusted relative HR (P compared with placebo)	Non-diabetic patients: adjusted relative HR (P compared with placebo)	P (difference in benefit between diabetic and nondiabetic patients)
Overall mortality	0.45 (P = .09)	0.94 (P = .55)	.04
Mortality from cardiovascular disorders	0.24 (P = .01)	0.87 (P = .37)	.02
Cardiovascular events	0.31 (P = .002)	0.74 (P = .02)	.01
Stroke	0.27 (P = .02)	0.62 (P = .02)	.13
Cardiac events	0.37 (P = .06)	0.79 (P = .10)	.12

Data from Tuomilehto J, Rastenyte D, Birkenhager WH, et al. Effects of calcium-channel blocker in older patients with diabetes and systolic hypertension. N Engl J Med 1999;340:680.

Similar trends were seen in patients who had diabetes in the SHEP trial (although benefits for total mortality and stroke did not reach statistical significance) [118] and in the Chinese trial on isolated systolic hypertension in the elderly [119]. Whether target BP less than 130/80 mm Hg (as is suggested in the JNC 7 guidelines for patients who have diabetes) is appropriate for the elderly remains to be determined. Some of the issues in choosing goal BPs are highlighted by Ames [120].

How well is treatment of hypertension tolerated in the elderly?

Side effects

Several large studies have demonstrated that treatment of elderly hypertensive patients can be accomplished with acceptable side-effect profiles and reasonably high compliance rates. The SHEP Pilot Study demonstrated compliance rates in excess of 80% even in patients over age 80 years [121], with no excess symptoms compared with placebo [107], although hypokalemia and hyperuricemia were more common. The European Working Party on High Blood Pressure in the Elderly reported that dry mouth, nasal stuffiness, and diarrhea were more common in treated (triamterene plus hydrochlorthiazide, with methyldopa added if needed to achieve target) patients, with methyldopa further increasing the likelihood of dry mouth and diarrhea. Treated patients were also more likely to develop hypokalemia, glucose intolerance, elevated creatinine and uric acid levels, and symptomatic gout [122,123]. Where possible, treatment regimens should be simplified, with the clinician mindful of the increasing risk of adverse drug reactions with increasing total number of medications ingested. In a study of 30,000 Medicare enrollees, diuretics were among the medications associated with an increased risk of preventable adverse drug events [124].

In a Department of Veterans Affairs Cooperative Study, 30% of patients achieved goal DBP in the placebo group at the end of 1 year, with the highest response rates in older white patients (38% compared with rates of 27% in older blacks and 23% in younger subjects). Discontinuation for exceeding the BP safety limits was twice as common in the placebo group. Discontinuation of study drug due to adverse effects, however, was higher in the placebo group (13%) compared with the active-treatment group (12%) [125].

In a small trial of middle-aged and elderly patients (average age, 68 years) who had systolic hypertension, Hollenberg and colleagues [126] reported that despite comparable lowering of BP with amlodipine and eplerenone, amlodipine was associated with a significant increase in ankle swelling, headache, facial flushing, constipation, and pronounced heart-beat, whereas eplerenone-treated patients had no significant new or worsening symptoms.

After controlling for baseline risk factors and adjustment for SBP as a time-dependent variable, Somes and coworkers [127] reported (SHEP trial) that in the active treatment arm only, a decrease in DBP of 5 mm Hg increased the risk of stroke (RR = 1.14, 95% CI: 1.05–1.22), coronary heart disease (RR = 1.08, 95% CI: 1.00–1.16), and cardiovascular disease (RR = 1.11, 95% CI: 1.05–1.16), with the effect beginning at DBP less than 65 mm Hg. This effect was seen in men and women, across the full spectrum of baseline disease status, and across all age groups (although small numbers of subjects aged >80 years led to a loss of statistical significance in that population).

Sexual dysfunction

Sexual dysfunction was prevalent in hypertensive men in the Treatment of Mild Hypertension Study (TOMHS). Age greater than 60 years and SBP greater than 140 mm Hg were associated with erectile problems at baseline. The study examined the association between five different medications and the presence of sexual dysfunction at 24 months of therapy, and found that chlorthalidone was associated with the highest incidence of erectile dysfunction (15.7% versus 4.9% in placebo). The other agents (amlodipine, acebutolol, doxazosin, and enalapril) had rates comparable to placebo [128].

Cognitive function and mood

Data are insufficient to determine whether aging affects the impact of antihypertensive agents on cognitive functioning. Muldoon and colleagues [129] reviewed the neuropsychologic consequences of antihypertensive medication use. Individual studies have reported adverse effects of certain β-blockers, nifedipine, reserpine, and diuretic therapy. Inconsistent findings between studies and methodologic differences, however, make it difficult to draw clinically meaningful conclusions. In the SHEP trial, active treatment of isolated systolic hypertension had no measured negative effects and, for some measures, a slight positive effect on cognitive, physical, and leisure function. There was no effect on measures related to emotional state [130]. As with any drug in the elderly, a temporal relationship between worsening cognition and the initiation of a new medication should prompt the clinician to evaluate the possibility of drug-induced cognitive dysfunction.

Dyslipidemia and other metabolic disruptions

Monane and coworkers [131] examined the New Jersey Medicaid and Medicare programs and found that elderly (65–99 years old) enrollees who were newly initiated on low-dose thiazide diuretic antihypertensive medications between 1981 and 1989 were not more likely to be subsequently started on a lipid-lowering agent, although users of high-dose thiazides (≥ 50 mg) had subsequent lipid-lowering therapy started nearly twice as often. Analysis of the SHEP trial (chlorthalidone first step) data revealed an insignificant increase in the development of new diabetes, although small effects on fasting glucose (+3.6 mg/dL, $P < .01$), total cholesterol (+3.5 mg/dL, $P < .01$), high-density lipoprotein (−0.77 mg/dL), creatinine (+0.03 mg/dL), triglycerides (+17 mg/dL), uric acid (+0.06 mg/dL), and potassium (−0.3 mmol/L) were observed [132].

Diabetes

Concern has been raised about the potential for β-blockers to attenuate the autonomic response, thereby increasing the risk of hypoglycemia. Shorr and colleagues [133] evaluated 13,559 elderly (mean age, 78 ± 7 years) participants in Tennessee's Medicaid program and found that there was no statistically significant increase or decrease in the risk of serious hypoglycemia among users of any class of antihypertensive agents compared with nonusers of antihypertensive drugs.

Accelerated hypertension

There have been multiple reports of adverse events related to precipitous drops in BP in patients with accelerated hypertension or hypertensive emergencies. Barring immediate life-threatening elevations of BP (eg, associated with acute ischemia), attempts should be made to lower BP over hours rather than over minutes, allowing time to reset the cerebral blood flow autoregulatory mechanisms. Because of the high prevalence of systolic hypertension and its attendant risk of cerebrovascular disease, elderly patients might be expected to be at higher risk of precipitous drops in BP. Although any agent that produces such a drop could provoke adverse effects, short-acting nifedipine has been singled out as a known culprit [134] and should be avoided in the elderly.

The very elderly

Although existing data demonstrate the risk associated with high BP and the benefits of treatment in the middle-aged and the "young old" (65–75 years), there is a growing body of data that suggests that it may be inappropriate to extrapolate these results to the very old (≥ 85 years). Vaitkevicius and coworkers [135] demonstrated that in frail elderly subjects 80 years and older, an aerobic exercise program is associated with a significant decline in resting SBP (146 ± 18 versus 133 ± 14 mm Hg, $P = .01$) and improves VO$_2$max. The Leiden 85 Plus study (mean age, 90 years), however, looked at all-cause mortality with a 5- to 7-year follow-up. Lower DBPs were associated with higher mortality rates, although most of this effect of low BP disappeared after controlling for multiple other risk factors [136]. After adjustment for age, sex, and baseline variables of health status, SBP (even >200 mm Hg) was not predictive of all-cause mortality, but DBP re-emerged as a predictor of cardiovascular mortality. In addition, Goodwin [137] pointed out that although the Framingham Heart Study found a positive linear relationship between BP and cardiovascular mortality in younger (35–64 years) and older (65–84 years) populations, when the sample is divided into 10-year increments, the positive association is seen only up to the 65- to 74-year age group. In the 75- to 84-year age group, SBP and DBP become inversely associated with cardiovascular mortality in men and women. In the Established Populations for Epidemiological Studies in the Elderly cohorts, in men, the positive relationship between SBP and survival persisted even after adjusting for age, functional status, medication use, medical diagnoses, and cognitive function. There was no relationship between BP and survival in women 85 years and older [138]. In the European Working Party on High Blood Pressure in the Elderly trial, the benefits of treatment were lost in patients over age 80 years [139,140].

Gueyffier and coworkers [141] conducted a meta-analysis of trials of hypertension in the elderly, limiting their analysis to data in patients over age 80 years. They found that treatment prevented 34% (95% CI: 8–52) of strokes. Although rates of major cardiovascular events and heart failure decreased 22% and 39%, respectively, there was no treatment benefit derived for cardiovascular death and a nonsignificant 6% (95% CI: −5 to 18) excess of death from all causes. Moreover, these investigators pointed out that the treatment benefits observed were not robust. "The addition of a single hypothetical trial of proper design (ad hoc power) with no treatment effect would be enough to make the results non-significant" [141].

To address the concerns raised from these studies and from epidemiologic information, the Hypertension in the Very Elderly Trial Working Group initiated a study in patients 80 years and older. Patients were allocated randomly to a diuretic-based regimen, to an ACE inhibitor–based regimen, or to no treatment. The calcium channel blocker diltiazem was added to these regimens as needed to achieve target BP control. Data from the open-design pilot study revealed a nonsignificant increase in mortality for the diuretic-based regimen (HR = 1.31, 95% CI: 0.75–2.27) and the ACE inhibitor–based regimen (HR = 1.14, 95% CI: 0.65–2.02). Fatal and nonfatal strokes were significantly reduced in the diuretic group (HR = 0.31, 95% CI: 0.12–0.79) but only insignificantly in the ACE inhibitor group (HR = −0.69, 95% CI: 0.30–1.31). Insignificant increases in cardiovascular, cardiac, and non–cardiovascular disease mortality were also noted despite (or perhaps because of) the 23/11–mm Hg drop in BPs in the active treatment groups. No significant differences in creatinine, potassium, or uric acid levels occurred in any group [142]. The larger trial has been designed as a randomized, blinded trail and is currently under way [143].

Summary

Hypertension is predictive of a wide variety of subsequent adverse events in elderly patients, at least up to the age of 80 years. Treatment can reduce these adverse outcomes, although the benefits in the very elderly remain somewhat unclear. In the very elderly, there appears to be a reduction in cardiovascular events, but this reduction is perhaps at the expense of an increase in overall mortality. Target BPs in the elderly remain controversial. Among patients who have not had previous stroke or significant cardiovascular or renal disease, the benefits of reducing the SBP below 159 mm Hg are well documented. There is some evidence to suggest, however, that if doing so increases the day–night difference in BP by more than 20% or is associated with a decline in DBP below 65 mm Hg, then the benefits of treatment may be attenuated or lost. In addition, there is some suggestion that reducing SBP consistently below 135 mm Hg may accelerate cognitive decline.

There appears to be a role for sodium restriction in those who can comply without otherwise compromising nutrient intake. Likewise, exercise may be beneficial and have benefits beyond simply lowering BP. Weight loss in those who are overweight may also help in lowering the BP. For most patients, low-dose thiazides such as hydrochlorothiazide are likely to be the appropriate first-line therapy (even in patients who have diabetes) unless they exacerbate or precipitate urinary incontinence or gout or complicate concomitant drug therapy (eg, lithium treatment of bipolar disorder). In very elderly patients, the apparent beneficial effects on strokes, major cardiovascular events, and heart failure rates may justify treating despite lack of benefit on overall mortality.

References

[1] American Heart Association, Learn and Live; Statistical Fact Sheet-Populations; Older Americans and Cardiovascular Disease Statistics. Available at: www.americanheart.org/downloadable/heart/1103832534191FS08OLD5.pdf. Accessed February 24, 2005.

[2] US Census Bureau, Decennial Census and Projections. Older Americans 2004: key indicators of wellbeing. Available at: www.aginstats.gov. Accessed February 24, 2005.

[3] Sohyoun NR, Lentzner H, Hoyeret D, et al. Trends in causes of death among the elderly. Aging Trends. No. 1. Hyatsville (MD): National Center for Health Statistics; 2001. Available at: www.cdc.gov/nchs/data/agingtrends/01death.pdf. Accessed February 24, 2005.

[4] McClellan W, Hall WD, Brogan D, et al. Isolated systolic hypertension: declining prevalence in the elderly. Prev Med 1987;16:686–95.

[5] Chobanian AV, Bakris GL, Balck HR, et al. The Seventh Report of the Joint National Committee on Prevention, Detection, Evaluation, and Treatment of High Blood Pressure. JAMA 2003;289:2560–72.

[6] Psaty BM, Furgerg CD, Kuller LH, et al. Isolated systolic hypertension and subclinical cardiovascular disease in the elderly. JAMA 1992;268:1287–91.

[7] Auseon A, Ooi WL, Hossain M, et al. Blood pressure behavior in the nursing home: implications for diagnosis and treatment of hypertension. J Am Geriatr Soc 1999;47: 285–90.

[8] Sagie A, Larson M, Levy D. The natural history of borderline isolated hypertension. N Engl J Med 1993;329:1912–7.

[9] Hakala SM, Tilvis RS. Determinants and significance of declining blood pressure in old age. Eur Heart J 1998;19:1872–8.

[10] Burt VL, Whelton P, Roccella EJ, et al. Prevalence of hypertension in the US adult population: results from the Third National Health and Nutrition Examination Survey, 1988–1991. Hypertension 1995;25:305–13.

[11] State-specific trends in self-reported blood pressure screening and high blood pressure— United States, 1991–1999. MMWR Morb Mortal Wkly Rep 2002;51(21):456–60.

[12] Egan BM, Lackland DT, Cutler NE. Awareness, knowledge, and attitudes of older Americans about high blood pressure. Arch Intern Med 2003;163:681–7.

[13] Franklin SS, Jacobs MJ, Wong ND, et al. Predominance of isolated systolic hypertension among middle-aged and elderly US hypertensives: analysis based on National Health and Nutrition Examination Survey (NHANES) III. Hypertension 2001;37(3):869–74.

[14] Hyman DK, Pavlik VN. Characteristics of patients with uncontrolled hypertension. N Engl J Med 2001;345(7):479–86.

[15] Gambassi G, Lapane K, Sgadari A, et al. Prevalence, clinical correlates, and treatment of hypertension in elderly nursing home residents. Arch Intern Med 1998;158:2377–85.

[16] Hajjar IM, Grim CE, Kotchen TA. Dietary calcium lowers the age-related rise in blood pressure in the United States: the NHANES III survey. J Clin Hypertens (Greenwich) 2003; 5(2):122–6.

[17] Hajjar IM, Grim CE, George V, et al. Impact of diet on blood pressure and age-related changes in blood pressure in the US population: analysis of NHANES III. Arch Intern Med 2001;161(4):589–93.

[18] Gurwitz JH, Avorn J, Bohn RL, et al. Initiation of antihypertensive treatment during nonsteroidal anti-inflammatory drug therapy. JAMA 1994;272:781–6.

[19] Johnson AG, Nguyed TV, Day RO. Nonsteroidal anit-inflammatory drugs may elevate blood pressure. Ann Intern Med 1994;121:289–300.

[20] Coates ML, Rembold CM, Farr BM. Pseudoephedrine did not increase blood pressure in hypertension. J Fam Pract 1995;40:22–6.

[21] Dinenno FA, Dietz NM, Joyner MJ. Aging and forearm postjunctional alpha-adrenergic vasoconstriction in healthy men. Circulation 2002;106(11):1349–54.

[22] Nash D, Magder L, Lustberg M, et al. Blood lead, blood pressure, and hypertension in perimenopausal and postmenopausal women. JAMA 2003;289:1523–32.

[23] Wilking AVB, Belanger A, Kannel WB, et al. Determinants of isolated systolic hypertension. JAMA 1988;260:3451–5.

[24] Scuteri A, Bos AJG, Brand LJ, et al. Hormone replacement therapy and longitudinal changes in blood pressure and postmenopausal women. Ann Intern Med 2001;135: 229–38.

[25] He J, Ogden LG, Vupputuri S, et al. Dietary sodium intake and subsequent risk of cardiovascular disease in overweight adults. JAMA 1999;282:2027–34.

[26] Strazzullo P, Iacone R, Iacoviello L, et al. Genetic variation in the renin-angiotensin system and abdominal adiposity in men: the Olivetti Prospective Heart Study. Ann Intern Med 2003;138:17–23.

[27] Nieto FJ, Herrington DM, Redline S, et al. Sleep apnea and markers of vascular endothelial function in a large community sample of older adults. Am J Respir Crit Care Med 2004; 169(3):354–60.

[28] Ancoli-Israel S, Gehrman P, Kripke DF, et al. Long-term follow-up of sleep disordered breathing in older adults. Sleep Med 2001;2(6):511–6.

[29] Lakatta E. Cardiovascular system. In: Masoro E, editor. Handbook of physiology, section 11. Aging. New York: Oxford University Press; 1995. p. 413–74.

[30] Fleg JL. Alterations in cardiovascular structure and function with advancing age. Am J Cardiol 1986;57:33C–44C.

[31] Vaitkevicius PV, Fleg JL, Engel JH, et al. Effects of age and aerobic capacity on arterial stiffness in healthy adults. Circulation 1993;88:1456–62.

[32] Smulyan S, Safar ME. The diastolic blood pressure in systolic hypertension. Ann Intern Med 2000;132:233–7.

[33] Berry KL, Cameron JD, Dart AM, et al. Large-artery stiffness contributes to the greater prevalence of systolic hypertension in elderly women. J Am Geriatr Soc 2004;52: 368–73.

[34] Pan HYM, Hoffman BB, Pershe RA, et al. Decline in beta adrenergic receptor-mediated vascular relaxation with aging in man. J Pharmacol Exp Ther 1986;239(3):802–7.

[35] Kawamoto A, Shimada K, Matsubayashi K, et al. Cardiovascular regulatory functions in elderly patients with hypertension. Hypertension 1989;13:401–7.

[36] Messerli FG, Glade LB, Dreslinski GR, et al. Hypertension in the elderly: haemodynamic, fluid volume and endocrine findings. Clin Sci 1981;61:393s–4s.

[37] Messerli FG, Sundgaard-Riise K, Ventura HO, et al. Essential hypertension in the elderly: haemodynamics, intravascular volume, plasma renin activity, and circulating catechol-amine levels. Lancet 1983;2(8357):983–6.

[38] Sowers JR, Mohanty PK. Effect of advancing age on cardiopulmonary baroreceptor function in hypertensive men. Hypertension 1987;10:274–9.

[39] Mukai S, Gagnon M, Iloputaife I, et al. Effect of systolic blood pressure and carotid stiffness on baroreflex gain in elderly subjects. J Gerontol 2003;58A(7):626–30.

[40] Kannel WB. Some lessons in cardiovascular epidemiology from Framingham. Am J Cardiol 1976;37:269–82.

[41] Sutton KC, Dai WS, Kuller LH. Asymptomatic carotid artery bruits in a population of elderly adults with isolated systolic hypertension. Stroke 1985;16(5):781–4.

[42] Vokonas PS, Kannel WB, Cupples LA. Epidemiology and risk of hypertension in the elderly: the Framingham Study. J Hypertens 1988;6(Suppl 1):S3–9.

[43] Staessen JA, Gasowski J, Wang JG, et al. Risks of untreated and treated isolated systolic hypertension in the elderly: meta-analysis of outcome trials. Lancet 2000;355:865–72.

[44] Alli C, Avanzini F, Bettelli G, et al. The long-term prognostic significance of repeated blood pressure measurements in the elderly. Arch Intern Med 1999;159:1205–12.

[45] Mattace-Raso FUS, van der Cammen TJM, van Popele NC, et al. Blood pressure components and cardiovascular events in older adults: the Rotterdam Study. J Am Geriatr Soc 2004;52:1538–42.

[46] Seshadri S, Wolf PA, Beiser A, et al. elevated midlife blood pressure increases stroke risk in elderly persons. Arch Intern Med 2001;161:2343–50.

[47] Haider AW, Larson MG, Franklin SS, et al. Systolic blood pressure, diastolic blood pressure, and pulse pressure as predictors of risk for congestive heart failure in the Framingham Heart Study. Ann Intern Med 2003;138:10–6.

[48] van der Meer IM, Iglesisa del Sol A, Hak AE, et al. Risk factors for progression of atherosclerosis measured at multiple sites in the arterial tree: the Rotterdam Study. Stroke 2003;34:2374–9.

[49] van Leeuwen R, Ikram MK, Vingerling JR, et al. blood pressure, atherosclerosis, and the incidence of age-related maculopathy: the Rotterdam Study. Invest Ophthalmol Vis Sci 2003;44:3771–7.

[50] Kuo HK, Sorond F, Iloputaife I, et al. Effect of blood pressure on cognitive functions in elderly persons. J Gerontol (Med Sci) 2004;59A(11):1191–4.

[51] Wallace RB, Lemke JH, Morris MC, et al. Relationship of free-recall memory to hypertension in the elderly. the Iowa 65+ Rural Health Study. J Chron Dis 1985;38(6): 475–81.

[52] Glynn RK, Beckett LA, Hebert LE. Current and remote blood pressure and cognitive decline. JAMA 1999;281:438–45.

[53] Petitti DB, Crooks VC, Buckwalter JG, et al. Blood pressure levels before dementia. Arch Neurol 2005;62:112–6.

[54] de Leeuw FE, de Groot JC, Oudkerk M, et al. Hypertension and cerebral white matter lesions in a prospective cohort study. Brain 2002;125:765–72.

[55] van Dijk EJ, Breteler MMB, Schmidt R, et al. The association between blood pressure, hypertension, and cerebral white matter lesions: Cardiovascular Determinants of Dementia Study. Hypertension 2004;44:625–30.

[56] Sacktor N, Gray S, Kawas C. Systolic blood pressure within an intermediate range may reduce memory loss in an elderly hypertensive cohort. J Geriatr Psychiatry Neurol 1999;12: 1–6.

[57] SHEP Cooperative Research Group. Prevention of Stroke by antihypertensive drug treatment in older persons with isolated systolic hypertension: final results of the Systolic Hypertension in the Elderly Program (SHEP). JAMA 1991;265:3255–65.

[58] Forette F, Seux ML, Staessen JA, et al. Prevention of dementia in randomized double-blind placebo-controlled Systolic Hypertension in Europe (Syst-Eur) trail. Lancet 1998;352: 1347–51.

[59] Forette F, Seux ML, Staessen JA, et al. The prevention of dementia with antihypertensive treatment: new evidence from the Systolic Hypertension in Europe (Syst-Eur) study. Arch Intern Med 2002;162(18):2046–52.

[60] in't Veld BA, Ruitenberg A, Hoffman A, et al. Antihypertensive drugs and incidence of dementia: the Rotterdam Study. Neurobiol Aging 2001;22:407–12.

[61] Drayer JIM, Weber MA, Deyoung JL, et al. Circadian blood pressure patterns in ambulatory hypertensive patients: effects of age. Am J Med 1982;73:493–9.

[62] Pasqualini R, Foroni M, Salvioli G, et al. The "nondipper" elderly: a clinical entity or a bias? J Am Geriatr Soc 2004;52:967–71.

[63] Kario K, Matsuo T, Kobayashi H, et al. Nocturnal fall of blood pressure and silent cerebrovascular damage in elderly hypertensive patients. Hypertension 1996;27: 130–5.

[64] Nakamura K, Oita J, Yamaguchi T. Nocturnal blood pressure dip in stroke survivors: a pilot study. Stroke 1995;26:1373–8.

[65] Cavallini MC, Roman MJ, Blank SG, et al. Association of the auscultatory gap with vascular disease in hypertensive patients. Ann Intern Med 1996;124:877–83.

[66] Hla KM, Feussner JR. Screening for pseudohypertension. Arch Intern Med 1988;148: 673–6.

[67] Bailey RH, Bauer JH. A review of common errors in the indirect measurement of blood pressure. Arch Intern Med 1993;153:2741–8.

[68] Hla KM, Vokaty KA, Feussner JR. Observer error in systolic blood pressure measurements in the elderly. Arch Intern Med 1986;146:2373–6.

[69] Bailey RH, Knaus VL, Bauer JH. Aneroid sphygmomanometers: an assessment of accuracy at a university hospital and clinics. Arch Intern Med 1991;151:1409–12.

[70] Smith NL, Psaty BM, Rutan GH, et al. The association between time since last meal and blood pressure in older adults: the cardiovascular health study. J Am Geriatr Soc 2003; 51(6):824–8.

[71] Kohara K, Jiang Y, Igase M, et al. Postprandial hypotension is associated with asymptomatic cerebrovascular damage in essential hypertensive patients. Hypertension 1999;33(1 Pt 2):565–8.

[72] Le Couteur DG, Fisher AA, Davis MW, et al. Postprandial systolic blood pressure responses of older people in residential care: association with risk of falling. Gerontology 2003;49(4):260–4.

[73] Ensrud KE, Nevitt MC, Yunis C, et al. Postural hypotension and postural dizziness in elderly women. The study of osteoporotic fractures. The Study of Osteoporotic Fractures Research Group. Arch Intern Med 1992;152(5):1058–64.

[74] Mukai S, Lipsitz LA. Orthostatic hypotension. Clin Geriatr Med 2002;18(2):253–68.

[75] Hossain M, Ooi WL, Lipsitz LA. Intra-individual postural blood pressure variability and stroke in elderly nursing home residents. J Clin Epidemiol 2001;54(5):488–94.

[76] Luukinen H, Koski K, Laippala P, et al. Orthostatic hypotension and the risk of myocardial infarction in the home-dwelling elderly. J Intern Med 2004;255(4):486–93.

[77] Masuo K, Mikami H, Ogihara T, et al. Changes in frequency of orthostatic hypotension in elderly hypertensive patients under medications. Am J Hypertens 1996;9(3):263–8.

[78] Vogt MT, Cauley JA, Newman A, et al. Decreased ankle/arm blood pressure index and mortality in elderly women. JAMA 1993;270:465–9.

[79] Sutton KC, Wolfson SK, Kuller LH. Carotid and lower extremity arterial disease in elderly adults with isolated systolic hypertension. Stroke 1987;18:817–22.

[80] Tuomilehto J. Body mass index and prognosis in elderly hypertensive patients: a report from the European Working Party on High Blood Pressure in the Elderly. Am J Med 1991; 90(Suppl 3A):34S–41S.

[81] Fagard R. Serum cholesterol levels and survival in elderly hypertensive patients: analysis of data from the European Working Party on High Blood Pressure in the Elderly. Am J Med 1991;90(Suppl 3A):62S–3S.

[82] Wachtell K, Insen H, Olsen MH, et al. Albuminuria and cardiovascular risk in hypertensive patients with left ventricular hypertrophy: the LIFE Study. Ann Intern Med 2003;139: 901–6.

[83] Staessen JA, Thijs L, Fagard R, et al. Predicting cardiovascular risk using conventional vs ambulatory blood pressure in older patients with systolic hypertension. JAMA 1999;282: 539–46.

[84] Wing LMH, Brown MA, Beilin LJ, et al. "Reverse white-coat hypertension" in older hypertensives. J Hypertens 2002;20:639–44.

[85] Kannel WB, Sorlie P, Gordon T. Labile hypertension: a faulty concept? Circulation 1980; 61(5):1183–7.

[86] Tsuji I, Imai Y, Nagai K, et al. Proposal of reference values for home blood pressure measurement prognostic criteria based on a prospective observation of the general population in Ohasama, Japan. Am J Hypertens 1997;10(4 pt 1):409–18.

[87] Hozawa A, Ohkubo T, Nagai K, et al. Prognosis of isolated systolic and isolated diastolic hypertension as assessed by self-measurement of blood pressure at home. Arch Intern Med 2000;160:3301–6.

[88] Hitzenberger G, Magometschnigg D. Blood pressure characteristics of hypertensive patients in Austria as determined by self-monitoring (SCREEN-II). Blood Press 2003; 12(3):134–8.

[89] Thijs L, Staessen JA, Celis H, et al. Reference values for self-recorded blood pressure. Arch Intern Med 1998;158:481–8.

[90] Turnbull SM, Magennis SP, Turnbull CJ. Patient self-monitoring of blood pressure in general practice: the 'inverse white-coat' response. Br J Gen Pract 2003;53(488):221–3.

[91] Cuspidi C, Michev I, Meani S, et al. Left ventricular hypertrophy in treated hypertensive patients with good blood pressure control outside the clinic, but poor clinic blood pressure control. J Hypertens 2003;21(8):1575–81.

[92] Thijs L. Age-related hypotensive effect of placebo and active treatment in patients older than 60 years. Am J Med 1991;90(Suppl 3A):24S–6S.

[93] Joossens JV, Kesteloot H. Trends in systolic blood pressure, 24-hour sodium excretion, and stroke mortality in the elderly in Belgium. Am J Med 1991;90(Suppl 3A):5S–11S.

[94] Niarchos AP, Weinstein DL, Laragh JH. Comparison of the effects of diuretic therapy and low sodium intake in isolated systolic hypertension. Am J Med 1984;77:1061–8.

[95] Kaplan NM. Electrolytes: their importance in hypertension in the elderly. Geriatr Cardiovasc Med 1988;1:123–7.

[96] Midgley JP, Mathew AG, Greenwood CM, et al. Effect of reduced dietary sodium on blood pressure. A meta-analysis of randomized controlled trials. JAMA 1986;275:1590–7.

[97] Geleijnse JM, Witteman JC, Bak AA, et al. Reduction in blood pressure with a low sodium, high potassium, high magnesium salt in older subjects with mild to moderate hypertension. BMJ 1994;309(6952):436–40.

[98] Luft FC, Weinberger MH, Fineberg NS, et al. Effects of age on renal sodium homeostasis and its relevance to sodium sensitivity. Am J Med 1987;82(Suppl 1B):9–15.

[99] Hoption Cann SA, van Netten JP, van Netten C. Iodized Salt and hypertension. Arch Intern Med 2002;162:104.

[100] Khaw KT, Barret CE. Dietary potassium and stroke-associated mortality: a 12-year prospective population study. N Engl J Med 1987;316:235–40.

[101] Whelton PK, He J, Cutler JA, et al. Effects of oral potassium on blood pressure. Meta-analysis of randomized controlled trials. JAMA 1997;277:1624–32.

[102] Applegate WB, Miller ST, Elam JT, et al. Nonpharmacologic intervention to reduce blood pressure in older patients with mild hypertension. Arch Intern Med 1992;152:1162–6.

[103] Whelton PK, Appel LJ, Espeland MA, et al. Sodium reduction and weight loss in the treatment of hypertension in older persons: a randomized Trial of Nonpharmacologic Interventions in the Elderly (TONE). JAMA 1998;279:839–46.

[104] Pearce LK, Engel BT, Burton JR. Behavioral treatment of isolated systolic hypertension in the elderly. Biofeedback Self Regul 1989;14(3):207–17.

[105] Jajich CL, Ostfeld AM, Freeman DH. Smoking and coronary heart disease mortality in the elderly. JAMA 1984;252:2831–4.

[106] Cushman WC, Khatri I, Materson BJ, et al. Treatment of hypertension in the elderly: III. Response of isolated systolic hypertension to various doses of hydrochlorthiazide—results of a Department of Veterans Affairs Cooperative Study. Arch Intern Med 1991;151: 1954–60.

[107] Hulley SB, Furberg CD, Gurland B, et al. Systolic Hypertension in the Elderly Program (SHEP): antihypertensive efficacy of chlorthalidone. Am J Cardiol 1985;56:913–20.

[108] Perry HM, Davis BR, Price TR, et al. Effect of treating isolated systolic hypertension on the risk of developing various types and subtypes of stroke. JAMA 2000;284:465–71.

[109] Kostis JB, Davis BR, Cutler J, et al. Prevention of heart failure by antihypertensive drug treatment in older persons with systolic hypertension. JAMA 1997;278:212–6.

[110] Bleumink BS, Deinum J, Mosterd A, et al. Antihypertensive treatment is associated with improved left ventricular geometry: the Rotterdam Study. Pharmacoepidemiol Drug Saf 2004;13:703–9.

[111] Schulman ST, Weiss JL, Becker LC, et al. The effects of antihypertensive therapy on left ventricular mass in elderly patients. N Engl J Med 1990;322:1350–6.

[112] Applegate W, Dismuke SE, Runyan JW. Treatment of hypertension in the elderly: a time for caution? J Am Geriatr Soc 1984;32:21–3.

[113] ALLHAT Officers and Coordinators for the ALLHAT Collaborative Research Group. The Antihypertensive and Lipid-Lowering Treatment to Prevent Heart Attack Trial. Major outcomes in high-risk hypertensive patients randomized to angiotensin-converting enzyme inhibitor or calcium channel blocker vs diuretic: the Antihypertensive and Lipid-Lowering Treatment to Prevent Heart Attack Trial (ALLHAT). JAMA 2002;288(23): 2981–97.

[114] Wing LM, Reid CM, Ryan P, et al. A comparison of outcomes with angiotensin-converting enzyme inhibitors and diuretics for hypertension in the elderly. N Engl J Med 2003;348: 583–92.

[115] Pahor M, Shorr RI, Somes GW, et al. Diuretic-based treatment and cardiovascular events in patients with mild renal dysfunction enrolled in the Systolic Hypertension in the Elderly Program. Arch Intern Med 1998;158:1340–5.

[116] Warram JH, Laffel LM, Valsania P, et al. Excess mortality associated with diuretic therapy in diabetes mellitus. Arch Intern Med 1991;151(7):1350–6.

[117] Tuomilehto J, Rastenyte D, Birkenhager WH, et al. Effects of calcium-channel blocker in older patients with diabetes and systolic hypertension. N Engl J Med 1999;340:677–84.

[118] Curb JD, Pressel SL, Cutler JA, et al. Effect of diuretic-based antihypertensive treatment on cardiovascular disease risk in older diabetic patients with isolated systolic hypertension. JAMA 1996;276:1886–92.

[119] Wang JG, Staessen JA, Gong L, et al. Chinese trial on isolated systolic hypertension in the elderly. Arch Intern Med 2000;160:211–20.
[120] Ames R. Goal blood pressure in treating hypertension. Arch Intern Med 2002;162:105–6.
[121] Black DM, Brand RJ, Greenlick M, et al. Compliance to treatment for hypertension in the elderly patients: the SHEP Pilot Study. J Gerontol 1987;42(5):552–7.
[122] Fletcher AE. Adverse treatment effects in the trial of the European Working Party on High Blood Pressure in the Elderly. Am J Med 1999;90(Suppl 3A):42S–4S.
[123] Staessen J. The Determinants and prognostic significance of serum uric acid in elderly patients of the European Working Party on High Blood Pressure in the Elderly Trial. Am J Med 1999;90(Suppl 3A):50S–4S.
[124] Field TS, Gurwitz JH, Harrold LR, et al. Risk factors for adverse drug events among older adults in the ambulatory setting. J Am Geriatr Soc 2004;52:1349–54.
[125] Preston RA, Materson BJ, Reda DJ, et al. Placebo-associated blood pressure response and adverse effects in the treatment in the treatment of hypertension. Arch Intern Med 2000; 160:1449–54.
[126] Hollenberg NK, Williams GH, Anderson R, et al. Symptoms and the distress they cause: comparison of an aldosterone antagonist and a calcium channel blocking agent in patients with systolic hypertension. Arch Intern Med 2003;163:1543–8.
[127] Somes GW, Pahor M, Shorr RI, et al. The role of diastolic blood pressure when treating isolated systolic hypertension. Arch Intern Med 1999;159:2004–9.
[128] Grimm RH, Grandits GA, Prineas RJ, et al. Sexual dysfunction in men was greater with chlorthalidone than with placebo, acebutolol, amlodipine, doxazosin or enalapril. Hypertension 1997;29:8–14.
[129] Muldoon MF, Waldstein SR, Jennings JR. Neuorpsychological consequences of antihypertensive medication use. Exp Aging Res 1995;21:353–68.
[130] Applegate WB, Pressel S, Wittes J, et al. Impact of the treatment of isolated systolic hypertension on behavioral variables. Results from the Systolic Hypertension in the Elderly Program. Arch Intern Med 1994;154(19):2154–60.
[131] Monane M, Gurwitz JH, Bohn RI, et al. The impact of thiazide diuretics on the initiation of lipid-reducing agents in older people: a population-based analysis. J Am Geriatr Soc 1997; 45:71–5.
[132] The Systolic Hypertension in the Elderly Program. Influence on long-term, low-dose, diuretic-based, antihypertensive therapy on glucose, lipid, uric acid, and potassium levels in older men and women with isolated systolic hypertension. Arch Intern Med 1998;158: 741–51.
[133] Shorr RI, Ray WA, Daugherty JR, et al. Antihypertensives and the risk of serious hypoglycemia in older persons using insulin or sulfonylureas. JAMA 1997;278:40–3.
[134] Grossman E, Messerli FH, Grodzicki T, et al. Should a moratorium be placed on sublingual nifedipine capsules given for hypertensive emergencies and pseudoemergencies? JAMA 1996;276:1328–31.
[135] Vaitkevicius PV, Ebersold C, Shah MS, et al. Effects of aerobic exercise training in community-based subjects aged 80 and older: a pilot study. J Am Geriatr Soc 2002;50(12): 2009–13.
[136] Boshuizen HC, Izaks GJ, van Buuren S, et al. Blood pressure and mortality in elderly people aged 85 and older: community based study. 1998;316:1780–4.
[137] Goodwin JS. Embracing complexity: a consideration of hypertension in the very old. J Gerontol 2003;58A(7):653–8.
[138] Satish S, Freeman DH Jr, Ray L, et al. The relationship between blood pressure and mortality in the oldest old. J Am Geriatr Soc 2001;49(4):367–74.
[139] Birkenhager AA, Broxko P, Bulpitt C, et al. Influence of antihypertensive drug treatment on morbidity and mortality in patients over the age of 60 years. European Working Party on High blood Pressure in the Elderly (EWPHE) results: subgroup analysis. J Hypertens Suppl 1986;4(6):S642–7.

[140] Birkenhager AA, Brixko R, Bulpitt C, et al. Efficacy of antihypertensive drug treatment according to age, sex, blood pressure, and previous cardiovascular disease in patients over the age of 60. Lancet 1986;2(8057):589–92.

[141] Gueyffier F, Bulpitt C, Boissel JP, et al. Antihypertensive drugs in very old people: a subgroup meta-analyisis of randomized controlled trials. Lancet 1999;353:793–6.

[142] Bulpitt CJ, Beckett NS, Cooke J, et al. Results of the pilot study for the Hypertension in the Very Elderly Trial. J Hypertens 2003;21:2409–17.

[143] Bulpitt C, Fletcher A, Beckett N, et al. Hypertension in the Very Elderly Trial (HYVET): protocol for the main trial. Drugs Aging 2001;18:151–64.

[144] Hansson L, Hedner T, Lund-Johansen P, et al. Randomised trial of effects of calcium antagonists compared with diuretics and β-blockers on cardiovascular morbidity and mortality in hypertension: the Nordic Diltiazem (NORDIL) study. Lancet 2000;356: 359–65.

[145] Hansson L, Lindhold LH, Ekbom T, et al. Randomised trial of old and new antihypertensive drugs in elderly patients: cardiovascular mortality and morbidity. The Swedish Trial in Old Patients with Hypertension-2 study. Lancet 1999;354:1751–6.

[146] Lindholm LH, Hansson L, Ekbom T, et al. Comparison of antihypertensive treatments in preventing cardiovascular events in elderly diabetic patients: results from the Swedish Trial in Old Patients with Hypertension-2. STOP Hypertension-2 Study Group. J Hypertens 2000;18(11):1671–5.

[147] Dahlof B, Lindholm LH, Hansson L, et al. Morbidity and mortality in the Swedish Trial in Old Patients with Hypertension. (STOP-Hypertension). Lancet 1991;338:1281–5.

[148] MRC Working Party. Medical Research Council trial of treatment of hypertension in older adults: principal results. BMJ 1992;304:405–12.

[149] Wing LM, Reid CM, Ryan P, et al. Second Australian National Blood Pressure Study (ANBP2). Australian comparative outcome trial of ACE inhibitor- and diuretic-based treatment of hypertension in the elderly. Management Committee on behalf of the High Blood Pressure Research Council of Australia. Clinical & Experimental Hypertension 1997;19(5–6):779–91.

ELSEVIER
SAUNDERS

Prim Care Clin Office Pract
32 (2005) 755–775

PRIMARY CARE:
CLINICS IN
OFFICE PRACTICE

Approaches to Appropriate Drug Prescribing for the Older Adult

Kim Petrone, MD[a,b,*], Paul Katz, MD, CMD[b]

[a]St. Ann's Community, 1600 Portland Avenue, Rochester, NY 14621, USA
[b]University of Rochester School of Medicine, Monroe Community Hospital,
435 East Henrietta Road, Rochester, NY 14620, USA

Persons over age 65 years represent the largest consumers of medications. Results of the Slone Epidemiologic Survey suggest that 94% of women over age 65 years living in the community take at least 1 medication and 12% take 10 or more medications [1]. This observation combined with the general aging of the population, the increased number of available medications, and the increased marketing of medications challenges the primary care physician's efforts to craft the optimal drug regimen for each older adult seen in the office. Chief among these challenges is achieving a balance between prescribing an untenable number of medications to address the many chronic conditions prevalent in this population and avoiding a sense of therapeutic nihilism and consequent denial of efficacious medications to elderly patients. To fully appreciate the enormity of this task, the physician must understand the

- Pharmacodynamic and pharmacokinetic changes that occur with age
- Rate of adverse reactions and drug–drug interactions in the elderly
- Evidence for use of particular medications in an elderly population
- Medications that have been deemed harmful to most older adults
- Use of over-the-counter medications and herbal preparations
- Financial constraints particular to this population that affect compliance

Pharmacokinetic and pharmacodynamic changes in the elderly

The pharmacokinetics of an orally administered drug refers to the rate at which it is absorbed, distributed, metabolized, and eliminated from the body. Aging has little effect on the absorption of most drugs, although there

---

* Corresponding author. Medical Administration, St. Ann's Community, 1600 Portland Avenue, Rochester, NY 14621.

E-mail address: KPetrone@StAnnsCommunity.com (K. Petrone).

doi:10.1016/j.pop.2005.06.011

may be a change in the rate of absorption in older persons taking many medications. Absorption of many floroquinolones, for example, can be impaired if taken concomitantly with iron.

Unlike absorption, drug distribution changes with age because of associated changes in body composition—namely, an increase in fat stores and a decrease in total body water [2]. As such, drugs that are water soluble (or hydrophilic) such as ethanol or lithium have a lower volume of distribution, whereas fat-soluble drugs (or lipohilic drugs) such as diazepam and trazadone have a larger volume of distribution. Practically speaking, this means that in an older population, hydrophilic drugs reach steady state quicker and are eliminated more expeditiously compared with lipophilic medications that require more time to reach steady state and are eliminated at a slower rate. Moreover, drugs that are highly protein bound, such as digoxin, often have a higher proportion of unbound, pharmacologically active drug in older persons because of decreases in albumin that can occur in association with many of the chronic conditions prevalent in an older population [2].

Metabolism of medications is affected by age because of an age-related decrease in hepatic blood flow and liver size. As such, drugs that undergo phase I reactions in the liver and are converted to active metabolites often accumulate in older persons. With a few exceptions, drugs that are conjugated in the liver and converted to inactive metabolites by way of phase II reactions involving glucuronidation and sulfate conjugation are thus preferred in this population. Examples of medicines undergoing phase I reactions include valium and amitriptyline; medicines undergoing phase II reactions include lorazepam and oxazepam. Drug elimination is also often reduced in the geriatric population because of reductions in renal blood flow, kidney size, and glomerular filtration that accompany many chronic conditions. It is important to recognize that serum creatinine is not an accurate reflection of creatinine clearance in this population. Because of the decrease in lean muscle mass and attendant decrease in creatinine production, normal serum creatinine values may be associated with a significant decline in renal function. As such, it is always prudent to estimate creatinine clearance by using the Cockroft-Gault equation or the modified diet in renal disease equation shown in Box 1.

The pharmacodynamics of a drug refers to the time course and intensity of the drug's effect. The pharmacodynamics of some drugs changes with age, with a tendency for older persons to experience a heightened effect. This increased sensitivity may be due to changes in the drug–receptor interactions, postreceptor events, or organ pathology that results from various chronic diseases that may accompany aging. The possible effects that aging may have on the pharmacodynamics of a few common drugs are listed in Table 1. Ultimately, the changes in pharmacodynamics and pharmacokinetics support the adage of "start low and go slow." It is prudent to initiate drugs at a low dosage and to titrate slowly to achieve the desired therapeutic benefit. For some medications (eg, lithium, digoxin, and

---

Box 1. Estimation of creatinine clearance

Cockroft-Gault equation for estimating creatinine clearance (Cr Cl):

$$\text{Cr Cl in milliliters per minute}^a = \frac{(140 - \text{age in years})(\text{weight in kilograms})}{72(\text{serum creatinine in milligrams per deciliter})}$$

[a]For women, this number should be multiplied by 0.85.

Modified diet in renal disease equation for estimating creatinine clearance:

$$\text{Cr Cl in milliliters per minute}^b = \exp(5.228 - 1.154 \times \log[\text{serum creatinine}]) - (0.203 \times \log[\text{age}])$$

[b]For women, this number should be multiplied by 0.742; for African Americans, this number should be multiplied by 1.21.

From Levey AS, Bosch JP, Lewis JB, et al. A more accurate method to estimate glomerular filtration rate from serum creatinine: a new prediction equation. Modification of Diet in Renal Disease Study Group. Ann Intern Med 1999;130:461–70; with permission.

---

some anticonvulsants), dosages for the older adult will remain low and still prove effective because of the aforementioned changes in pharmacokinetics and pharmacodynamics, whereas for other medications (eg, angiotensin-converting enzyme inhibitors and some serotonin selective reuptake inhibitor antidepressants), slow titration to doses typically used in a younger population may be more appropriate [2].

Adverse drug reactions, drug–drug interactions, and drug–disease interactions in the elderly

Adverse drug reactions are common primarily because of the age-associated alterations in pharmacokinetics and pharmacodynamics and the sheer number of medications prescribed for older persons. Recent estimates suggest that 35% of ambulatory older adults experience an adverse drug reaction on a yearly basis and 29% require evaluation by a physician or evaluation in the emergency room/hospital for the adverse reaction. If ranked as a disease, adverse drug reactions would be the fifth leading cause

Table 1
Effects of aging on selected medications: changes in pharmacodynamics

Drug	Action	Effect of aging
Morphine	Acute analgesic effect	Increase
Albuterol	Bronchodilation	Decrease
Glyburide	Chronic hypoglycemic effect	No change
Diazepam	Sedation	Increase
Furosemide	Latency and size of peak diuretic response	Decrease
Nitroglycerin	Venodilation	No change

Data from Beers M, Berkow R. The Merck manual of geriatrics: clinical pharmacology. 3rd edition. Whitehouse Station (NJ): Merck Research Laboratory; 2000.

of death in America. Costs of medication-related problems in the ambulatory setting alone are estimated to surpass $75 billion [3].

Although much has been published about these reactions in the long-term care and acute care setting, little has been known until recently about the types of adverse drug reactions common in the outpatient setting. In 2003, Gurwitz and colleagues published a review of the frequency and potential prevention of adverse drug reactions in an outpatient population receiving care through a Medicare choice plan [4]. In a 1-year period in which 27,617 enrollees were followed, 1523 adverse drug events were identified. Of these events, 38% were categorized as serious, life-threatening, or fatal; 27% were considered preventable. Unlike the long-term care setting in which psychotropic medications have been identified as prime culprits, most preventable events in this outpatient population were related to cardiovascular medications followed by diuretics, nonopioid analgesics, hypoglycemics, and anticoagulants. The investigators concluded that the generalization of their results to the current population of Medicare enrollees translates into 1.9 million adverse drug events each year and approximately 180,000 life-threatening adverse drug reactions per year, of which about 50% would be preventable [4].

How can providers reduce the number of adverse drug reactions? The study by Gurwitz and colleagues [4] suggested that the largest number of preventable adverse reactions occurred at the prescribing or monitoring stages. Prescribing errors included wrong drug choices, wrong dose choices, inadequate patient education, and prescription of a drug for which there was a well-established, clinically important interaction with another drug. Monitoring errors included inadequate laboratory evaluation of drug therapies and failure to respond to signs, symptoms, or laboratory evidence of drug toxicity. Moreover, this failure to respond to evidence of drug toxicity may have been underestimated by the study, considering that such signs and symptoms may be atypical in older persons or poorly reported in those suffering from chronic cognitive impairments. Ultimately, the investigators postulated that in addition to physician education, health care systems need to respond to this problem by (1) making information on adverse drug reactions more accessible to patients, (2) enhancing the surveillance and reporting of adverse drug reactions, and (3) using computerized physician order entry, which could alert providers of possible drug–drug interactions, inappropriate doses, and the need for laboratory monitoring with particular drugs [4].

Another way to prevent adverse drug reactions in the older population is to make providers conscious of the prescribing cascade. This cascade is often initiated by an adverse drug reaction that is misinterpreted by the provider as a new medical condition. Such a misdiagnosis may result in a prescription for an additional and unnecessary medication, thus increasing the risk for further adverse drug reactions and drug–drug interactions [5]. Examples of such cascades include the use of dopamine agonists to treat neuroleptic-induced parkinsonism and the prescription of antihypertensive medications to treat elevations in blood pressure caused by nonsteroidal anti-inflammatory drugs [6]. Results of a case-control study of geriatric patients enrolled in the New Jersey Medicaid program support this notion. The study showed that elderly patients using nonsteroidal anti-inflammatory drugs had an odds ratio of 1.66 for being placed on an antihypertensive compared with those not using these analgesics. Even more impressive, the odds ratio of being placed on a medication for parkinsonism was 5.2 for those who were prescribed 20 mg or more of metoclopramide compared with those not receiving this medication [5].

A final important concept in relation to adverse drug reactions in the elderly is the notion of drug–disease interactions. Because the burden of chronic illnesses increases with age, persons over age 65 years are at higher risk for experiencing such drug–disease interactions. Examples of such interactions include increased sensitivity or paradoxic reactions to psychotropic medications in persons who have dementia or worsening of urinary retention in men who have benign prostatic hypertrophy when an anticholinergic medication is prescribed (Table 2). In addition, the consequences of adverse drug reactions may be more serious in older persons because of the burden of their comorbidities. A younger person who falls due to excess sedation from a medication is less likely to have a hip fracture, whereas an older woman with osteoporosis is at substantial risk for this untoward outcome [7].

Zhan and colleagues [8] suggested in their recently published article on potentially harmful drug–drug and drug–disease interactions that prescribers may not fully attend to these issues. Using data obtained from the National Ambulatory Medical Care Survey and the National Hospital Medical Care Survey from 1995 to 2000, these investigators found that for visits in which two or more prescriptions were written, 0.76% of the visits resulted in inappropriate drug–drug combinations. Moreover, 2.58% of visits in which a prescription was written resulted in an inappropriate drug–disease combination. The most common inappropriate drug–drug interactions included those in which a medication that might interact negatively

Table 2
Selected drug–disease interactions in the elderly

Disease	Drug	Potential adverse outcome
Benign prostatic hypertrophy	α-agonists, anticholinergics	Urinary retention
Dementia	Anticholinergics, benzodiazepine	Increased confusion
Hypertension	Nonsteroidal anti-inflammatory drugs	Increased blood pressure
Parkinson's disease	Antipsychotics	Worsening of movement disorder
Osteoporosis	Corticosteroids	Fracture
Constipation	Anticholinergics, opiates, calcium channel blockers	Worsening of constipation
Diabetes	Corticosteroids	Hyperglycemia
Renal impairment	Nonsteroidal anti-inflammatory drugs, radiocontrast dye	Renal failure
Venous insufficiency	Dihydropyridine calcium channel blockers	Increased lower extremity edema

with warfarin was added to the medication regimen; the most common drug–disease interactions included the prescription of anticholinergic medications, bethanacol, or narcotics to men who had benign prostatic hypertrophy. The most significant predictor of having an inappropriate combination prescribed was the sheer number of medications prescribed, again underscoring the need to carefully weigh the risk/benefit ratio of each medication [8]. Examples of drug–drug interactions are listed in Table 3.

Elderly population and drug trials: toward an evidence-based geriatric practice

Although much has been written about adverse drug reactions in the elderly, there is a relative dearth of studies looking at the efficacy of medications in an older population, making it even more difficult for the clinician to intelligently weigh the potential benefit and risk of pharmacologic therapy. Despite the fact that older people represent the fastest growing segment of the population, they are often systematically excluded from clinical studies. Bugeja and colleagues [9], for example, reviewed all original research articles published in major British medical journals (including the *British Medical Journal, Gut, Lancet,* and *Thorax*) from 1996 to 1997 and found that roughly 33% of the articles excluded persons 75 years and older without justification. Lee and colleagues [10] reviewed the inclusion of persons 75 years and older in randomized controlled trials of cardiovascular interventions for acute coronary syndrome from 1966 to 2000 and found that this group was grossly under-represented. Between 1966 and 1990, this group accounted for only 2% of all patients enrolled. This number increased to only 13% in studies recruiting patients after 1995, despite the fact that this age

Table 3
Selected clinically important drug–drug interactions in the elderly

Drug	Interacting drug	Mechanism	Effect
Digoxin	Amiodarone	Decreased renal or nonrenal clearance of digoxin	Digitalis toxicity
	Verapamil		
	Dilitiazem		
Warfarin	Metronidazole	Inhibition of drug metabolism	Increased anticoagulation
	Omeprazole		
	Trimethoprim-sulafmethoxazole		
Levothyroxine	Calcium carbonate	Levothyroxine adsorbs calcium carbonate in an acidic environment	Reduced T_4 absorption
			Increased thyrotropin levels [29]
Diuretic	Nonsteroidal anti-inflammatory drugs	Decreased renal perfusion	Renal impairment
Acetylcholinesterase inhibitor	Anticholinergic medications	Decreased ability to favorably augment acetylcholine level	Potentially less effective as a therapy for dementia [30]

Data from Beers M, Berkow R. The Merck manual of geriatrics: clinical pharmacology. 3rd edition. Whitehouse Station (NJ): Merck Research Laboratory; 2000.

group represented approximately 37% of patients hospitalized for a myocardial infarction and about 60% of all deaths attributable to myocardial infarctions. Although there are many postulated underpinnings for this exclusion, including fears about adverse drug reactions, drug–drug and drug–disease interactions, and poor compliance, none seems to justify the current state of ageist exclusion. To help mitigate this problem, the Food and Drug Administration issued guidelines to enhance the participation of older persons in clinical trials in 1989 and, more recently in 1997, began requiring drug companies to include a separate geriatric-use section in their drug labeling [11]. The most recent legislation, however, falls short of requiring drug companies to perform additional studies in older persons and, thus, the ability of providers to truly embrace an evidenced-based approach in their prescribing patterns remains limited at best.

Faced with little direct evidence on the efficacy of medications in the older population, clinicians often extrapolate and apply the data obtained from studies performed in a younger cohort to their geriatric patients. This practice may result in significant iatrogenesis; for example, in the SHOCK ("should we emergently revascularize occluded coronaries for cardiogenic shock?") trial, it was found that persons under age 70 years who were suffering from cardiogenic shock had a survival benefit if revascularization of the coronary arteries was pursued over a more conservative approach.

Applying these data to an older population over age 70 years, however, would not be clinically prudent because the trial also found that the older cohort seemed to fare better when the conservative approach was adopted over revascularization. Although treatment and medication regimens certainly need to be individualized, the current state of applying data from a younger population to older adults is fraught with problems [10].

Instead of applying data obtained from a younger cohort to older patients, clinicians may become overly cautious or even nihilistic and adopt a prescribing strategy that ignores potentially beneficial therapies in response to the lack of research applicable to this population. In the last decade, several studies have alleged that there is gross undertreatment of older persons with therapies that have been substantiated by the medical literature to improve outcomes [11]. Sloane and colleagues [12], for example, examined medication regimens of 2014 persons over age 65 years residing in assisted living facilities and found that 62% of persons who had congestive heart failure were not receiving an angiotensin-converting enzyme inhibitor, 51% of patients who had osteoporosis were not receiving calcium supplementation, and 37% were not receiving any antiplatelet or anticoagulant treatment despite a history of a cerebrovascular attack. Of the people who had a history of coronary artery disease, only 40% were receiving aspirin and only 34% were receiving a β-blocker. These numbers are comparable to the numbers found in studies enrolling community-dwelling seniors. Bungard and coworkers [13], for example, conducted a literature review of all studies examining the use of angiotensin-converting enzyme inhibitors in community-dwelling persons who had congestive heart failure and found that the two patient characteristics most associated with the lack of use of an angiotensin-converting enzyme inhibitor were female sex and older age. Andrade and colleagues [14] found that secondary prevention for osteoporotic fractures in a group of community-dwelling women was grossly underprescribed, with only 24% receiving any medication treatment in the year following the fracture. Of interest, increasing age was among the most robust predictors of not receiving such therapy.

Beers Criteria: applicability to an ambulatory population

Although recent critiques of provider prescribing styles have focused on the denial of potentially beneficial therapies, the earliest efforts at improving prescribing for a senior population focused on heightening provider awareness of the medications to avoid in an older population. The first of these publications appeared in 1991 and explicitly identified medications that were potentially inappropriate to use in frail older adults residing in nursing homes. This set of criteria, now known as the Beers Criteria, was agreed on by a consensus panel comprising experts from geriatric medicine, psychiatry, and pharmacology. Medications on this list were categorized as potentially inappropriate for use because of limited effectiveness or because they posed a high risk for adverse effects. Among the drugs included were long half-life benzodiazepines and hypoglycemics, drugs with significant anticholinergic activity, and analgesic preparations containing propoxyphene [15]. This list was updated in 1997 and again in 2002 to (1) include new products and scientific information; (2) ascertain the generalizability of the list to all persons over age 65 years (regardless of functional level or place of residence); and (3) assign a relative rating of severity for potential adverse outcomes for each of the cited medications. The newest iteration of this list classifies medications into two broad headings, including 48 medications or medication classes that should generally be avoided in persons over age 65 years and 20 medications that should not be used in older persons known to have specific conditions (Table 4) [3].

In the years following the initial publication of the Beers Criteria, several studies were published that linked use of these medications to poor health outcomes [16]. Fick and colleagues [3], for example, found that ambulatory seniors who were prescribed a medication from the Beers Criteria list were more likely to be hospitalized or evaluated in an emergency room than those not taking such a medication. Chin and colleagues found poor control of pain and worse physical functioning in persons prescribed a medication from the list [16,17]. Despite these studies, Zhan and colleagues [18] found that the number of outpatient prescriptions for these medications remains unacceptably high. Using data from the 1996 Medical Expenditure Survey, these authors found that 21% of community-dwelling elderly persons were receiving a potentially inappropriate medication as defined by the Beers Criteria. Moreover, they noted that elderly women, persons who had poor health, and those with a lengthy medication list were the most likely recipients of these medications. It is unfortunate that the most recent data published by Goulding and coworkers in 2004 suggests that little has changed since 1996 [16]. Using data from the National Ambulatory Medical Care Survey and the National Hospital Medical Care Survey, these investigators examined the rate of inappropriate medication prescriptions to older persons from 1995 through 2000. They found that rates of prescription of inappropriate medications in the outpatient realm did not appreciably change over this period and noted that three drugs (propoxyphene, amitriptyline, and diazepam) represented the bulk of the inappropriate prescriptions. Like earlier studies, this study found that elderly women were more likely to receive these medications compared with their male counterparts [16].

Barriers to compliance

Further complicating the issue of drug prescribing in the elderly is compliance. Medication compliance in this population is influenced by a host of factors: the number of medications, common sensory impairments, cognitive impairments, functional impairments, and limitations in financial resources. This last factor may be a more important barrier than many

Table 4

2002 Criteria for potentially inappropriate medication use in older adults: independent of diagnoses or conditions

Drug	Concern	Severity rating (high or low)
Propoxyphene (Darvon) and combination products (Darvon with ASA, Darvon-N, and Darvocet-N)	Offers few analgesic advantages over acetaminophen, yet has the adverse effects of other narcotic drugs.	Low
Indomethacin (Indocin and Indocin SR)	Of all available nonsteroidal anti-inflammatory drugs, this drug produces the most CNS adverse effects.	High
Pentazocine (Talwin)	Narcotic analgesic that causes more CNS adverse effects, including confusion and hallucinations, more commonly than other narcotic drugs. Additionally, it is a mixed agonist and antagonist.	High
Trimethobenzamide (Tigan)	One of the least effective antiemetic drugs, yet it can cause extrapyramidal adverse effects.	High
Muscle relaxants and antispasmodics: methocarbamol (Robaxin), carisoprodol (Soma), chlorzoxazone (Paraflex), metaxalone (Skelaxin), cyclobenzaprine (Flexeril), and oxybutynin (Ditropan). Do not consider the extended-release Ditropan XL	Most muscle relaxants and antispasmodic drugs are poorly tolerated by elderly patients, since these cause anticholinergic adverse effects, sedation, and weakness. Additionally, their effectiveness at doses tolerated by elderly patients is questionable.	High
Flurazepam (Dalmane)	This benzodiazepine hypnotic has an extremely long half-life in elderly patients (often days), producing prolonged sedation and increasing the incidence of falls and fracture. Medium-or short-acting benzodiazepines are preferable.	High
Amitriptyline (Elavil), chlordiazepoxide-amitriptyline (Limbitrol), and perphenazine-amitriptyline (Triavil)	Because of its strong anticholinergic and sedation properties, amitriptyline is rarely the antidepressant of choice for elderly patients.	High

Table 4 (*continued*)

Drug	Concern	Severity rating (high or low)
Doxepin (Sinequan)	Because of its strong anticholinergic and sedating properties, doxepin is rarely the antidepressant of choice for elderly patients.	High
Meprobamate (Miltown and Equanil)	This is a highly addictive and sedating anxiolytic. Those using meprobamate for prolonged periods may become addicted and may need to be withdrawn slowly.	High
Doses of short-acting benzodiazepines: doses greater than lorazepam (Ativan), 3 mg; oxazepam (Serax), 60 mg; alprazolam (Xanax), 2 mg; temazepam (Restoril), 15 mg; and triazolam (Halcion), 0.25 mg	Because of increased sensitivity to benzoadiazepines in elderly patients, smaller doses may be effective as well as safer. Total daily doses should rarely exceed the suggested maximums.	High
Long-acting benzodiazepines: chlordiazepoxide (Librium), chlordiazepoxide-amitriptyline (Limbitrol) clidinium-chlordiazepoxide (Librax), diazepam (Valium), quazepam (Doral), halazepam (Paxipam), and chlorazepate (Tranxene)	These drugs have a long half-life in elderly patients (often several days), producing prolonged sedation and increasing the risk of falls and fractures. Short- and intermediate-acting benzodiazepines are preferred if a benzodiazepine is required.	High
Disopyramide (Norpace and Norpace CR)	Of all antiarrhythmic drugs, this is the most potent negative inotrape and therefore may induce heart failure in elderly patients. It is also strongly anticholinergic. Other antiarrhythmic drugs should be used.	High
Digoxin (Lanoxin) (should not exceed >0.125 mg/d except when treating atrial arrhythmias)	Decreased renal clearance may lead to increased risk of toxic effects.	Low
Short-acting dipyridamole (Persantine). Do not consider the long-acting dipyridamole (which has better properties than the short-acting in older adults) except with patients with artificial heart valves	May cause orthostatic hypotension.	Low

(*continued on next page*)

Table 4 (*continued*)

Drug	Concern	Severity rating (high or low)
Methyldopa (Aldomet) and methyldopa-hydrochlorothiazide (Aldoril)	May cause bradycardia and exacerbate depression in elderly patients.	High
Reserpine at doses >0.25 mg	May induce depression, impotence, sedation, and orthostatic hypotension.	Low
Chlorpropamide (Diabinese)	It has a prolonged half-life in elderly patients and could cause prolonged hypoglycemia. Additionally, it is the only oral hypoglycemic agent that causes SIADH.	High
Gastrointestinal antispasmodic drugs: dicyclomine (Bentyl), hyoscyamine (Levsin and Levsinex), propantheline (Pro-Banthine), belladonna alkaloids (Donnatal and others), and clidinium-chlordiazepoxide (Librax)	GI antispasmodic drugs are highly anticholinergic and have uncertain effectiveness. These drugs should be avoided (especially for long-term use).	High
Anticholinergics and antihistamines: chlorpheniramine (Chlor-Trimeton), diphenhydramine (Benadryl), hydroxyzine (Vistaril and Atarax), cyproheptadine (Periactin), promethazine (Phenergan), tripelennamine, dexchlorpheniramine (Polaramine)	All nonprescription and many prescription antihistamines may have potent anticholinergic properties. Nonanticholinergic antihistamines are preferred in elderly patients when treating allergic reactions.	High
Diphenhydramine (Benadryl)	May cause confusion and sedation. Should not be used as a hypnotic, and when used to treat emergency allergic reactions, it should be used in the smallest possible dose.	High
Ergot mesyloids (Hydergine) and cyclandelate (Cyclospasmol)	Have not been shown to be effective in the doses studied.	Low
Ferrous sulfate >325 mg/d	Doses >325 mg/d do not dramatically increase the amount absorbed but greatly increase the incidence of constipation.	Low
All barbiturates (except phenobarbital) except when used to control seizures	Are highly addictive and cause more adverse effects than most sedative or hypnotic drugs in elderly patients.	High

Table 4 (*continued*)

Drug	Concern	Severity rating (high or low)
Meperidine (Demerol)	Not an effective oral analgesic in doses commonly used. May cause confusion and has many disadvantages to other narcotic drugs.	High
Ticlopidine (Ticlid)	Has been shown to be no better than aspirin in preventing clotting and may be considerably more toxic. Safer, more effective alternatives exist.	High
Ketorolac (Toradol)	Immediate and long-term use should be avoided in older persons, since a significant number have asymptomatic GI pathologic conditions.	High
Amphetamines and anorexic agents	These drugs have potential for causing dependence, hypertension, angina, and myocardial infarction.	High
Long-term use of full-dosage, longer half-life, non–COX-selective NSAIDs: naproxen (Naprosyn, Avaprox, and Aleve), oxaprozin (Daypro), and piroxicam (Feldene)	Have the potential to produce GI bleeding, renal failure, high blood pressure, and heart failure.	High
Daily fluoxetine (Prozac)	Long half-life of drug and risk of producing excessive CNS stimulation, sleep disturbances, and increasing agitation. Safer alternatives exist.	High
Long-term use of stimulant laxatives: bisacodyl (Dulcolax), cascara sagrada, and Neoloid except in the presence of opiate analgesic use	May exacerbate bowel dysfunction.	High
Amiodarone (Cordarone)	Associated with QT interval problems and risk of provoking torsades de pointes. Lack of efficacy in older adults.	High
Orphenadrine (Norflex)	Causes more sedation and anticholinergic adverse effects than safer alternatives.	High
Guanethidine (Ismelin)	May cause orthostatic hypotension. Safer alternatives exist.	High
Guanadrel (Hylorel)	May cause orthostatic hypotension.	High

(*continued on next page*)

Table 4 (*continued*)

Drug	Concern	Severity rating (high or low)
Cyclandelate (Cyclospasmol)	Lack of efficacy.	Low
Isoxsurpine (Vasodilan)	Lack of efficacy.	Low
Nitrofurantoin (Macrodantin)	Potential for renal impairment. Safer alternatives available.	High
Doxazosin (Cardura)	Potential for hypotension, dry mouth, and urinary problems.	Low
Methyltestosterone (Android, Virilon, and Testrad)	Potential for prostatic hypertrophy and cardiac problems.	High
Thioridazine (Mellaril)	Greater potential for CNS and extrapyramidal adverse effects.	High
Mesoridazine (Serentil)	CNS and extrapyramidal adverse effects.	High
Short acting nifedipine (Procardia and Adalat)	Potential for hypotension and constipation.	High
Clonidine (Catapres)	Potential for orthostatic hypotension and CNS adverse effects.	Low
Mineral oil	Potential for aspiration and adverse effects. Safer alternatives available.	High
Cimetidine (Tagamet)	CNS adverse effects including confusion.	Low
Ethacrynic acid (Edecrin)	Potential for hypertension and fluid imbalances. Safer alternatives available.	Low
Desiccated thyroid	Concerns about cardiac effects. Safer alternatives available.	High
Amphetamines (excluding methylphenidate hydrochloride and anorexics)	CNS stimulant adverse effects.	High
Estrogens only (oral)	Evidence of the carcinogenic (breast and endometrial cancer) potential of these agents and lack of cardioprotective effect in older women.	Low

Abbreviations: CNS, central nervous system; COX, cyclooxygenase; GI, gastrointestinal; NSAIDs, nonsteroidal anti-inflammatory drugs; SIADH, syndrome of inappropriate antidiuretic hormone secretion.

From Fick DM, Cooper JW, Wade WE, et al. Updating the Beers Criteria for potentially inappropriate medication use in older adults. Results of a US Consensus Panel of Experts. Arch Intern Med 2003;163:2719–20; with permission.

prescribers appreciate. Presently, seniors pay 42% of the nation's bill for prescription drugs, and the congressional budget office estimates that the average Medicare beneficiary will spend $3155 in the year 2006 on prescription drugs [11]. This number is staggering when one considers that the median household income for seniors is $23,000 [19]. The Medicare Prescription Drug Improvement and Modernization Act of 2003 was enacted in part to address the financial hurdle for older adults, yet opponents of the proposal warn that it may do little to change the significant financial barriers encountered by those over 65 years old. The act, which will take full effect in January 2006, represents the most sweeping change in Medicare legislation since its inception in 1965 [20]. It employs what many have termed a "doughnut design," providing 75% coverage for drug costs up to $2250 and paying 95% of costs over $5100. The "hole in the doughnut" refers to the lack of coverage for drug costs between these two dollar amounts for which beneficiaries will be responsible for 100% of the discounted cost. Thus, for an average beneficiary, there will be monthly premiums amounting to about $35, an annual deductible of $250, 25% of the next $2000 in drug costs, 100% of the next $2850, and 5% of costs over $5100. Low-income seniors are eligible for discounted premiums and will not be required to pay for drug costs falling in the "doughnut hole," but qualifying for this low-income status will require seniors to fall below 135% of the poverty level and possess less than $10,000 in assets. This coverage may represent a less substantial benefit than was previously available under state Medicaid programs for some low-income seniors, who will be required to forfeit this former benefit if they enroll in the Medicare program [20,21].

Leaving the debate about the relative value of the Medicare prescription plan aside, there is still much that prescribers can do to ease the financial burden incurred by this segment of the population. Remaining sensitive to financial constraints and choosing generic options are critical practices for clinicians who treat geriatric patients. A recent survey of primary care physicians in Massachusetts, however, suggests that there is significant room for improvement on both of these fronts. Glickman and colleagues [22] surveyed 132 primary care physicians to examine their awareness of the affordability of medications, the use of generic alternatives, and their level of understanding of drug costs. They found that although 85% of respondents reported that inability to afford medications was a problem for some of their patients, 20% did not believe generic brands were as safe or effective as their more expensive brand-name alternatives and 30% reported that they rarely or never accessed information on the cost of medications. An overwhelming majority of these physicians also underestimated the costs of most drugs. This apparent lack of knowledge about costs may not only adversely affect compliance on an individual-patient basis but also speaks to growing concerns about aggregate costs for drugs and health care at large.

Use of complementary medicine and over-the-counter medications in the elderly

As if overseeing prescription medications for an elderly population is not daunting enough, the clinician must also be mindful of older adults' use of herbal preparations and over-the-counter medications. The last decade has seen an enormous increase in the use of complementary medicine including herbal supplements. Although early studies suggested that the use of such therapy was more common in younger persons, Astin [23] found that persons over age 65 years were just as likely to use complementary medicine as their younger counterparts. In a follow-up study of complementary medicine use exclusively in an older population enrolled in a managed Medicare program, these investigators found that 24% of seniors used an herbal medicine. *Ginkgo biloba* extract, garlic, and ginseng were among the most common herbs used. Also of great importance was the study's finding that a majority (58%) of those using herbal supplements did not report this use to their primary care physicians, raising the risk for drug–herb interactions such as the interactions of ginkgo and garlic with drugs that increase an individual's risk for bleeding (Table 5) [24,25].

Over-the-counter medications also complicate prescribing for older adults. Recent reviews suggest that the average number of over-the-counter medications taken by seniors on a daily basis is about 1.8, with the highest usage in white Midwestern women [26]. The most commonly used over-the-counter medications in the over-65-year-old population include analgesics, with about 20% to 30% of older persons using such medications on any given day [27]. More than 60% of older people cannot identify the active ingredient in the over-the-counter pain remedy that they are taking, and 40% believe that these medications are too weak to cause any real harm [27]. This notion often leads to an omission on the part of the senior in relaying their usage of over-the-counter medications. Thus, it is imperative that the physician query their older patient on their use of nonprescription drugs.

Table 5
Selected drug–herb interactions

Drug	Interaction
Warfarin	Garlic, ginkgo, ginger, and feverfew may augment the anticoagulant effect; ginseng may decrease the effectiveness of warfarin
Nonsteroidal anti-inflammatory drugs	Gossypol and uva-ursi may add to gastrointestinal irritation
Levothyroxine	Horseradish and kelp may suppress thyroid function
Iron	Chamomile, feverfew, and Saint-John's-wort may inhibit iron absorption
Diuretics	Dandelion and uva-ursi may offset the antihypertensive effects of diuretics; gossypol may exacerbate hypokalemia
Digoxin	Hawthorne may potentiate effects; Siberian ginseng may interfere with assay

Data from Miller LG. Herbal medicinals: selected clinical considerations. Focusing on known or potential drug–herb interactions. Arch Intern Med 1998;158(20):2200–11.

Practical strategies

Although there are numerous important considerations involved in prescribing for the elderly, there are some practical strategies that can help providers successfully address this difficult yet common task. Foremost is the forging of a partnership with patients to better understand their health care goals in the context of prognosis and advance care directives. The topic of shared decision making is addressed in more detail in an article by Brody elsewhere in this issue. For patients who have a poor prognosis, for example, efforts at primary prevention with costly medications may be much less important than simply focusing efforts on symptom relief. This aspect of prescribing is also covered in the article by Ogle and Hopper elsewhere in this issue. In persons with multiple comorbidities who would require a significant, perhaps untenable number of medications based on published guidelines, this partnership will enable appropriate prioritization of medications. The partnership would also enable physicians to introduce patients to the concept of a time-limited trial of a medication. Such a trial enables providers to discuss with their patients the anticipated benefits of a particular drug therapy, the possible harm associated with the drug, and a proposed timeline for reviewing whether the benefits have been achieved and whether the benefits are worth the potential risks. If no ostensible benefit has been noted or if the potential side effects are not deemed tolerable for the described benefit, then the medication can be discontinued or changed to an alternate therapy.

Although counting medications is clearly not the best strategy for dealing with the challenges inherent to prescribing for the elderly, reviewing the medication list at every visit is crucial. This practice enables the physician to alter the list based on changes in health status, the addition of other medications, and the outcomes of any time-limited trials. Reviewing the medication list also provides an opportunity to review drugs prescribed by other providers (and any over-the-counter or herbal preparations) and to entertain the notion of medication discontinuation in light of changes in health status. Common scenarios in which medication weaning may be appropriate are listed in Box 2. Finally, reviewing medication lists serves as a reminder to order laboratory testing to monitor drug therapy; to reconsider less expensive, generic alternatives; and to review potential drug–drug and drug–disease interactions.

Periodically, the older patient should also be asked to bring in all medication bottles rather than a simple list. Reviewing medications in this fashion may reveal previously unrecognized problems with medication compliance because the number of pills remaining in each container or in the pill box can be assessed. By having the older patient review how and why he or she takes each medication, the physician can also determine whether compliance is being restricted by functional limitations (eg, arthritic changes of the hands making it difficult to open the container), sensory impairments

---

Box 2. Common clinical scenarios in which medication weaning could be considered

1. Situations in which an exclusive comfort care approach has been adopted but the individual is still receiving medication aimed at primary and secondary prevention
2. "Forgotten" steroids in patients stabilized from a previous exacerbation of chronic obstructive pulmonary disease, rheumatoid arthritis, or a remote history of polymyalgia rheumatica
3. Proton pump inhibitors initiated as prophylaxis during an acute care admission in persons without another indication for continuation of these medicines
4. Oral hypoglycemics after a person has been initiated on insulin
5. Newly diagnosed adverse events including delirium, falls, or orthostatic hypotension
6. Longstanding psychoactive medication with unclear target symptoms

---

From Brazeau S. Polypharmacy and the elderly. Can J Cont Med Educ 2001;2: 85–95.

(eg, inability to see the label on pill container or hear physician or pharmacist instructions), or cognitive impairments (making it difficult to comply with the regimen without supervision or assistance).

When initiating a medication, the clinician should start with the lowest feasible dose to achieve the desired effect. The clinician should seek data to support the drug's efficacy in older adults, bearing in mind that advanced age in and of itself should never be seen as a contraindication to potentially beneficial therapy. Clinicians should be aware of the prescribing cascade mentioned earlier and be certain that the medication being considered is not in response to an adverse drug reaction, a drug–drug interaction, or a drug–disease interaction.

Ultimately, the prescriber may embrace the "SEA-squared" model (Box 3). The safety of the medication should be considered by reviewing untoward outcomes revealed in drug trials and postmarketing clinical experience. The soundness of the proposed treatment should be considered in the context of the patient's prognosis and expressed goals for care. The efficacy or discernible benefit of the medication should be considered in the context of a structured scientific study, and more important, the putative effectiveness or the benefit of the medication should be assessed in the context of the patient's total environment. The appropriateness of the

---

Box 3. The SEA-squared model for evaluating prudent prescribing

Safety: is the medication safe based on clinical trials and clinical experience?

Soundness: is the medication in keeping with the patient's goals for care?

Effective: has the medication been shown to have a positive outcome in clinical trials?

Efficacious: will the medication prove beneficial in the "real world"?

Appropriate: is the medication approved for this indication? Would its use be consistent with the current standard of care?

Affordability: can the patient afford the medication?

---

medication should carefully be reviewed, taking into account regulatory approval by the Food and Drug Administration, scientific research, and the current standard of care. Finally, the affordability of the medication should be considered.

On a larger scale, the health care system should evolve in a manner that makes the challenge of prescribing for this age group less daunting. Demanding further research on particular therapies in this population, evaluating drug regimens over longer periods, and designing drug trials that include quality of life and functional outcomes will collectively attenuate the current challenge. Integrating possible drug–drug interactions in a unified, easily accessible database; working consistently in multidisciplinary teams in which a pharmacist can give real-time advice to prescribers; and computerized entry, which can immediately warn of problematic prescribing, will also significantly ease the prescriber's burden. Ultimately, prescribing medications for an older population may require a paradigm shift in how clinicians approach medical care. Optimal prescribing may require us to abandon the disease model, given its inherent tendency to cause the clinician to perceive patients as collections of maladies, each of which obligates a list of medications. In older persons, this model often leads to the prescription of an untenable number of medications that, in aggregate, have a dubious impact on the total well-being of the person or, worse yet, completely ignore the primary concerns of the patient, harm the patient, or force the patient to abandon beneficial therapies. In place of the disease model, we should adopt what Tinetti and Fried [28] have termed the *integrated individually tailored model of care*, whereby patients' priorities for their health care are paramount and medications are prescribed after careful consideration in accordance with these directives.

Summary

When prescribing for the older adult, the office-based physician walks the fine line between introducing the drugs that are considered best practices for each disease that the person has and acknowledging that as the number of drugs increases, the risks of adverse drug reactions, drug–drug interactions, or drug–disease interactions increase considerably. Establishing the clinician–patient partnership to develop goals of care is the first step in the process. Avoiding drugs that are likely to be associated with adverse outcomes (the Beers Criteria list) is an important next step, as is awareness of the prescribing cascade. It is also important, however, to not be overly pessimistic. Quality of care and quality of life may be greatly enhanced by careful use of prescription and over-the-counter medications in the older adult.

References

[1] Kaufman D, et al. Recent patterns of medication use in the ambulatory adult population of the United States. The Slone Survey. JAMA 2002;287(3):337–44.
[2] Semla T, Rochon P. Pharmacotherapy. In: Cobbs EL, Duthie EH, editors. Geriatrics Review Syllabus: a core curriculum in geriatric medicine. 5th edition. Malden (MA): Blackwell Publishing.
[3] Fick DM, Cooper JW, Wade WE, et al. Updating the Beers criterion for potentially inappropriate medication use in older adults: results of the US Consensus Panel of Experts. Arch Intern Med 2003;163(22):2716–24.
[4] Gurwitz JH, et al. Incidence and preventability of adverse drug events among older persons in the ambulatory setting. JAMA 2003;289(9):1107–16.
[5] Rochon PA, Gurwitz JH. Optimising drug treatment for elderly people. The prescribing cascade. BMJ 1997;315(7115):1096–9.
[6] Rochon PA, Gurwiz JH. Drug therapy. Lancet 1995;346:32–6.
[7] Crome P. What is different about older people? Toxicology 2003;192:49–54.
[8] Zhan C, Correa-de-Araujo R, Bierman AS, et al. Suboptimal prescribing in elderly outpatients: potentially harmful drug-drug interactions and drug-disease interactions. J Am Geriatr Soc 2005;53:262–7.
[9] Bugeja G, Kumar A, Arup K. Exclusion of elderly people from clinical research: a descriptive study of published reports. Br Med J 1997;315(7115):1059–61.
[10] Lee PY, Alexander KP, Hammill BG, et al. Representation of elderly persons and women in published randomized trials of acute coronary syndromes. JAMA 2001;286(6):708–13.
[11] Gurwitz JH. Polypharamcy: a new paradigm for quality drug therapy in the elderly? Arch Intern Med 2004;164(18):1957–69.
[12] Sloane PD, Gruber-Baldini A, Zimmerman S, et al. Medication undertreatment in assisted living settings. Arch Intern Med 2004;164(18):2031–7.
[13] Bungard T, Mc Alister F, Johnson J. Underutilization of ACE inhibitors in patients with congestive heart failure. Drugs 2001;61(14):2021–33.
[14] Andrade SE, Majumdar SR, Chan KE, et al. Low frequency of treatment of osteoporosis among postmenopausal women following a fracture. Arch Intern Med 2003;163(17):2052–7.
[15] Beers MH. Explicit criterion for determining potentially inappropriate medication use by the elderly. An update. Arch Intern Med 1997;157(14):1531–6.
[16] Goulding MR. Inappropriate medication prescribing for elderly ambulatory care patients. Arch Intern Med 2004;164(3):305–12.

[17] Chin MH, Wang LL, Jin L, et al. Appropriateness of medication selection for older persons in an urban academic emergency department. Acad Emerg Med 1999;6:1232–42.

[18] Zhan C, Sangl J, Bierman A, et al. Potentially inappropriate medications use in community dwelling elderly: findings from the 1996 Medical Expenditure Survey. JAMA 2001;286(22): 2823–9.

[19] Altman D. The new medicare prescription drug legislation. N Engl J Med 2004;350:9–10.

[20] Iglehart JK. The new medicare prescription drug benefit. N Engl J Med 2004;350:826–33.

[21] Emmer S, Allendorf L. The Medicare Prescription Drug Improvement and Modernization Act of 2003. J Am Geriatr Soc 2004;52:1013–5.

[22] Glickman L, Bruce EA, Caro FG, et al. Physicians' knowledge of drug costs in the elderly. J Am Geriatr Soc 1994;42(9):992–6.

[23] Astin JA. Why patients use alternative medicine. Results of a national study. JAMA 1998; 279(19):1548–53.

[24] Astin JA, Pelletier KR, Marie A. Complementary and alternative medicine use among elderly persons: one year analysis of a Blue Shield Medicare supplement. J Gerontol Med Sci 2000;55A(1):M4–9.

[25] Miller LG. Herbal medicinals: selected clinical considerations. Focusing on known or potential drug-herb interactions. Arch Intern Med 1998;158(20):2200–11.

[26] Hanlon JT, Fillenbaum GG, Ruby CM. Epidemiology of over-the-counter drug use in community dwelling elderly. United States perspective. Drugs Aging 2001;18(2):123–31.

[27] Roumie CL, Griffin MR. Over the counter analgesics in older adults: a call for improved labelling and consumer education. Drugs Aging 2004;21(8):485–98.

[28] Tinetti ME, Fried T. The end of the disease era. Am J Med 2004;116:179–85.

[29] Sing N, Sing PN, Hershman JM, et al. The effect of calcium carbonate on absorption of levothyroxine. JAMA 2000;283:2822–5.

[30] Carnahan RM, Lund BC, Perry PJ, et al. The concurrent use of anticholinergic and cholinesterase inhibitors: rare event or common practice? J Am Geriatr Soc 2004;52(12): 2082–7.

ELSEVIER
SAUNDERS

Prim Care Clin Office Pract
32 (2005) 777–792

PRIMARY CARE:
CLINICS IN
OFFICE PRACTICE

Depression in the Older Adult

Larry Lawhorne, MD

Department of Family Practice, Geriatric Education Center of Michigan,
College of Human Medicine, Michigan State University, B 215 West Fee Hall,
East Lansing, MI 48824, USA

Depression is the prototype of mood disorders in the older adult and can be defined as a painful emotional experience characterized by loss of interest or pleasure in life sufficient to affect function [1]. Depression, however, is not a single clinical entity. The depressive disorders listed in the *Diagnostic and Statistical Manual of Mental Disorders,* 4th edition (DSM-IV) [2] (Appendix 5b of this issue) are distinguished from one another based on a host of symptoms and signs. Conventional wisdom suggests that these disorders are common among older patients encountered in the primary care setting and that they are responsive to treatment. Challenging this conventional wisdom is a study conducted in the Netherlands that focuses on the natural history of late-life major depression, subthreshold depression, and dysthymic disorder. The study's findings suggest that DSM affective disorders are relatively rare in older adults and that outcomes are poor [3]. In contrast to major depression, clinically significant depressive symptoms that affect function and quality of life are frequent, leading some experts to question the usefulness of DSM criteria when assessing older adults [4].

Further complicating diagnostic considerations is another set of challenges for the primary care provider who evaluates and manages older patients. Do depressive symptoms represent major depression, minor or subthreshold depression, or dysthymia; or do such symptoms reflect loneliness, boredom, or fear? Are the depressive symptoms seen in the older office patient the consequence of a coexisting medical condition, change in residence, or neuropsychiatric condition other than depression? Where does bereavement fit into the evaluation?

Even more challenging is the difficult task of differentiating depressive disorders from the natural disengagement and withdrawal that may occur near the end of life, perhaps prompting cynics to say that "it's hard

E-mail address: larry.lawhorne@hc.msu.edu

doi:10.1016/j.pop.2005.06.001
primarycare.theclinics.com

to die without an SSRI [selective serotonin reuptake inhibitor]." Some have asserted that we have already tipped too far in the direction of "biomedicalizing" the aging process [5]. Depression and depressive symptoms are not caused by aging but are associated with the chronic illnesses, functional disabilities, and other losses that are more prevalent among older adults.

This article discusses the recognized risk factors and prevalence of depression and depressive symptoms in the older adult. Emerging evidence supporting the role that subcortical ischemic changes play in the development of late-life depression is presented [6]. Bereavement is addressed briefly, but bipolar disorders are not covered. A systematic process for the recognition and evaluation of depressive symptoms in the office setting is proposed, and a practical approach to treatment and monitoring is described. A guiding principle for treatment and monitoring is that pharmacotherapy without sufficient attention to nondrug interventions is unlikely to be successful.

Prevalence

A clear understanding of the prevalence of depressive disorders in older adults may help to dispel the myth that depression is an inevitable consequence of aging while raising awareness that certain segments of the older population are at substantial risk. The prevalence of depression or depressive symptoms in older adults depends on which segment of the population is studied. In general, major depression and depressive symptoms increase in frequency depending on whether the sample is drawn from the community, the physician's office, the hospital, or the nursing facility.

Community surveys suggest that the prevalence of major depression ranges from 1% to 4% [7]. The prevalence is higher among women, but there is no compelling evidence for significant racial or ethnic differences [7]. By contrast, 8% to 16% of community-dwelling elders who are interviewed exhibit clinically important depressive symptoms [7]. Among older adults who visit a primary care physician, 5% to 10% have major depression, whereas up to one third may have depressive symptoms [7,8]. Major depression affects 10.7% of African Americans and 10.9% of whites receiving home care services [9].

Major depression is seen in 10% to 12% of older adults who are sick enough or injured enough to be hospitalized, whereas an additional 23% have depressive symptoms [7]. Twelve percent to 20% of older adults living in nursing facilities have major depression, and another 35% experience important depressive symptoms [7,10].

Given this information about prevalence and accepting that 5% to 10% of older adults who visit the primary care provider may have a DSM depressive disorder, how should case finding be conducted? Some experts contend that screening in primary care is critical because of the high prevalence of depression and the high frequency of associated suicidal ideation [7]. The questions of whom to screen and how to screen are addressed in more detail after a review of risk factors.

Risk factors

Risk factors for late-life depressive disorders and depressive symptoms are traditionally divided into the psychosocial, the spiritual, and the biologic. Each of these categories has a rich and extensive literature, some of which is confusing or even contradictory. A few salient features are presented here, however, with the caveat that the office-based clinician who cares for the older adult with multiple medical conditions or multiple losses must maintain a high index of suspicion for depression.

Longitudinal cohort studies of well-defined populations have identified a number of important psychosocial risk factors for late-life depression: life events and ongoing difficulties, death of a spouse or other loved one, disability and functional decline, and lack of social support or contact [11]. Many older adults have one or more of these psychosocial risk factors yet do not develop depression. Reasons for this observation are that the psychosocial risk factors can be mitigated by personal or environmental factors [11]. In particular, the cognitive appraisal of a stressor and the processes whereby an older adult copes with or adapts to the stressor may determine whether he or she develops a depressive disorder [1]. Religious practice is associated with less depression at the individual level and among large groups of older adults, leading some to view "religious coping" as an important mechanism that buffers the effect of a number of risk factors for depression [7].

Among the biologic factors, genetic susceptibility (or family history) does not appear to be as important in the development of late-life depression as it does in younger individuals [7,12]. Rekindled interest in vascular depression, however, may direct attention to the genetic polymorphisms and mutations that are associated with specific vascular lesions in the central nervous system that are seen in greater numbers when comparing older adults who have late-life depression with those who are not depressed [7]. Other than genetic susceptibility, biologic risk factors for depression that have been considered include endocrine dysfunction, especially disturbance of the hypothalamic-pituitary-adrenal axis; immune system activation (inflammation); and nutritional deficiencies [7,12]. Although there is an abundance of literature addressing these biologic risk factors and their correlation with late-life depression, little is known about causal relationships [12].

A number of chronic medical conditions and certain medications have been implicated as risk factors for depression or depressive symptoms in older adults (Box 1) [1]. In the office setting, depression can be expected to occur in a substantial proportion of patients who have had a recent myocardial infarction, coronary artery bypass surgery, or stroke and among

Box 1. Common medical conditions and medications associated with depression

Cardiovascular conditions
Cardiovascular disease
Postmyocardial infarction
Postcoronary artery bypass surgery
  Cardiomyopathy (congestive or other)

Endocrine disorders
Thyroid (hyper- and hypothyroidism, thyroiditis)
Parathyroid (hyper- and hypoparathyroidism)
Adrenal (Cushing's and Addison's diseases)
Disorders of insulin secretion
Hypopituitarism

Metabolic or nutritional disorders
Hypokalemia or hyperkalemia
Hyponatremia or hypernatremia
Hypocalcemia or hypercalcemia
Hypomagnesemia
Metabolic acidosis or alkalosis
Hypoxemia
Vitamin deficiencies (B vitamins, folate)

Neurologic diseases
Parkinson's disease
Stroke
Alzheimer's disease
Subdural hematoma
Amyotrophic lateral sclerosis
Temporal lobe epilepsy
Multiple sclerosis
Normal-pressure hydrocephalus

Cancer
Brain tumors (primary or secondary)
Pancreatic cancer
Lung cancer (oat cell)
Bone metastases with hypercalcemia

Miscellaneous
End-stage renal disease (especially with uremia)
Hepatic failure with encephalopathy
Anemia

Infections (particularly viral)
Chronic pain

Medications
Central nervous system drugs
  Benzodiazepines
  Alcohol
  Levodopa
  Amantadine
  Major tranquilizers
  Stimulants (rebound)
Antihypertensives
  β-blockers
  Clonidine
  Reserpine
  Methyldopa
  Prazosin
  Guanethidine
Chemotherapuetic drugs
  Vincristine
  L-asparaginase
  Interferon
  Tamoxifen
Steroids
  Prednisone
  Estrogen preparations
Anticonvulsants
  Procarbazine
  Diphenylhydantoin
Others
  Cimetidine
  Digitalis
  Nonsteroidal anti-inflammatory drugs

Data from Koenig HG, Blazer DG. Depression, anxiety, and other mood disorders. In: Cassel CK, Leipzig RM, Cohen HJ, et al, editors. Geriatric medicine: an evidence-based approach. 4th edition. New York: Springer-Verlag; 2003. p. 1168, 1171.

those who have dementia, Parkinson's disease, renal insufficiency, or cancer [1,7,13]. In addition, because benzodiazepines and antihypertensive drugs are prescribed frequently in the office setting, health care practitioners should maintain a high index of suspicion for the development of depressive symptoms among patients who receive them.

The role of vascular risk factors in the etiology of late-life depression has been suggested for over 40 years but has received renewed attention with the widespread use of MRI of the brain [7]. Anatomic location and laterality of MRI signal hyperintensities in patients who have late-life depression may cause sufficient disruption in neural pathways to adversely affect mood and psychomotor state [6,14]. Two longitudinal studies have shown a positive relationship between vascular burden and the depressive symptoms over time [15,16]. The first study reported on 100 consecutive patients initially assessed while in a geriatric rehabilitation unit, followed by assessments for depression 6 and 18 months later [15]. Patients who had two or three cardiovascular risk factors demonstrated more depressive symptoms at 6- and 18-month follow-up assessments than patients who had one or no cardiovascular risk factors [15]. The second study reported on a cohort of 181 very old patients entering the independent-living section of a continuing care retirement community in which baseline depression was predictive of subsequent cardiovascular events [16].

Many of the demographic, psychosocial, and spiritual risk factors discussed earlier cannot be modified; however, vascular risk factors and the consequences of some medical conditions are at least partially modifiable [17], which may be advantageous when considering management of the older adult with late-life depression.

Bereavement

Bereavement is a natural and expected part of every older person's life experience. It is characterized by sensations of somatic distress and preoccupation with images of the deceased [1]. For an older adult, the death of a spouse appears to be associated with depressive symptoms and increased mortality [18]. The impact of losing a spouse, however, may be influenced by whether the surviving spouse had been a caregiver. Among individuals who are caregivers and already strained before the death of a spouse, the death does not appear to increase distress, whereas non-caregivers who lose a spouse experience an increase in depressive symptoms and weight loss [19].

Although grief is not a psychiatric illness, it can sometimes be associated with intense feelings of hopelessness, worthlessness, or suicidal ideation [1]. Many experts recommend that if an older adult meets DSM-IV criteria for major depression 2 months after the event that precipitated bereavement, he or she should be treated [1]. This approach, however, can be challenged, as suggested by the article on end-of-life care by Ogle and Hopper found elsewhere in this issue.

Recognition of late-life depression

How do health care professionals recognize depression in the primary care setting? Certainly, patients who have the risk factors described previously should attract attention, but should all older adults undergo screening? If so, which screening tests should be used?

The US Preventive Services Task Force gives a level B recommendation to screening for depression in adults, so long as systems are in place to ensure accurate diagnosis, effective treatment, and appropriate follow-up [20]. The Center for Epidemiologic Studies–Depression Scale and the Geriatric Depression Scale were found to have excellent properties in screening for major depression in 130 older primary care patients in three internal medicine practices using the Structured Clinical Interview for *Diagnostic and Statistical Manual of Mental Disorders*, 3rd edition, revised as the "gold standard" [21]. In a study involving 50 family physicians and 1580 adults (not just older adults), however, physicians performed poorly in identifying the 13.4% of patients who had major depression using the Center for Epidemiologic Studies–Depression Scale as a stand-alone measure or as a supplement to physician detection [22]. Performing the Center for Epidemiologic Studies–Depression Scale or the Geriatric Depression Scale is time-consuming. Given that a typical office visit includes three problems and eight care decisions [23], time is a scarce commodity, and briefer screening methods are preferable [24]. A positive answer to either of the following two questions is very sensitive and can identify more than 90% of patients who have major depression [25]:

- Have you often been bothered by feeling down, depressed, or hopeless?
- Have you often been bothered by little interest or pleasure in doing things?

The two-question screen, however, has a specificity of only 60% and requires additional testing to confirm [24].

A reasonable approach to recognition is to suspect a depressive disorder in any older adult with multiple medical conditions, stroke, neurodegenerative processes such as Alzheimer's disease or Parkinson's disease, or any of the psychosocial risk factors mentioned earlier. After suspicion is raised, the primary care provider should proceed with the evaluation described in the next section. An equally acceptable approach is to administer the two-question screen periodically on all older adults in the practice, followed by the evaluation described in the next section if either question generates a positive response.

Establishing the diagnosis

After depression is suspected, what are the next steps in the process? At least three of the symptoms on the list of DSM-IV criteria for major depression (weight loss, anorexia, and fatigue) are so general that they could be associated with a multitude of medical and neuropsychiatric conditions; therefore, a thorough history and physical examination are mandatory. Particular attention should be directed to previous similar episodes, drug or alcohol abuse, and thoughts of suicide [1]. As with the physical examination of persons with suspected dementia, the neurologic examination is crucial, looking for lateralization, tremor, changes in muscle tone, and slowed reflexes [1]. Generally recommended laboratory tests include complete blood count, chemistries, thyroid studies, and vitamin B_{12} level (methylmalonic acid and homocystine levels if vitamin B_{12} is in the low-normal range) [1]. A brain imaging study (CT or MRI) is indicated if there is an abnormal neurologic examination [1] or if vascular depression is suspected [7].

Following the history and physical examination and concurrent with the laboratory evaluation described earlier, DSM-IV criteria for the most commonly encountered depressive disorders can be applied. To establish a diagnosis of major depression, the person must have depressed mood or marked loss of interest that is experienced most of the day, nearly every day during at least 2 weeks, and of sufficient intensity to impair function. At least four of the following eight symptoms must also be present: (1) weight loss or anorexia, (2) sleep disturbance, (3) psychomotor agitation or retardation, (4) fatigue or loss of energy, (5) feelings of worthlessness or guilt, (6) diminished concentration, (7) thoughts of suicide, or (8) loss of interest, including decreased sexual interest [2]. Minor depression (also called subthreshold or subsyndromal depression) can be described as "near misses" for meeting DSM-IV criteria for major depression, whereas dysthymia is a chronic depression lasting 2 years or longer, again not fulfilling the criteria for major depression [7]. Making the diagnosis of minor depression is important because there is evidence that antidepressants can be effective [1].

Three other conditions should be considered when attending older adults with depressive symptoms: adjustment disorder with depressed mood, mood disorder caused by general medical condition, and substance-induced mood disorder. The first may be seen with retirement or following an ill-advised or undesired change of residence, the second as a direct physiologic effect of a medical diagnosis such as hypothyroidism, and the third as a consequence of problems such as alcohol abuse [1]. A single, validated screening question for problem drinking is: "When was the last time you had more than X drinks in one day?" where X equals 5 for men and 4 for women and possible responses are never, in the past 3 months, or over 3 months ago [26]. A positive response is "in the past 3 months" and requires a more detailed interview [24,26]. Patients who respond with "never" have only a 1% risk of problem drinking [24].

With the evaluation completed, the primary care provider should have a better understanding of what the depressive symptoms suggest in the individual older patient seeking office care. In addition, there should be a good grasp of coexisting medical and other neuropsychiatric conditions. Armed with this information, individualized treatment can be crafted that focuses on optimal management of medical and concomitant neuropsychiatric illnesses, help and referrals to address psychosocial and spiritual issues, and consideration of appropriate psychotherapeutic interventions and pharmacotherapy.

Treatment

The first step in treating the older adult with depression is initiating a plan to keep the person safe, which means asking about suicidal thoughts and about plans that the person may have to carry out suicide. If the person has thought about ending his or her life, then interventions to prevent suicide must be implemented, including eliciting help from family members and friends to remove weapons or stockpiles of drugs [1,27]. Suicide rates are higher in later life than in younger age groups [1]. Suicide risk factors include being a widow or widower, living alone, having a poor perception of health status, having sleep disturbance, not having someone to confide in, and having had recent stressful financial or interpersonal events [7]. White males are at greatest risk, especially when depression coexists with another mental illness or in the presence of alcohol abuse or dependence [1].

Education about depressive symptoms and the DSM depressive disorders is the next step [27]. A substantial proportion of the current cohort of older adults may view depression as a weakness of character or moral fiber and, therefore, reject the possibility of such a diagnosis. The older adult who has depression and his or her significant others need to understand that depression is the consequence of the biologic and psychosocial risk factors described previously and that targeted interventions can improve mood, function, and quality of life.

After safety measures are in place to minimize the chance of successful suicide (eg, removal of stockpiled medications or weapons) and education about depression has been initiated, basic supportive activities should be offered. The office staff can be pivotal in successful supportive activities by listening, by being empathetic, by mobilizing appropriate family and community resources, and by arranging spiritual support. Findings from a randomized controlled trial involving 12 primary care practices and comparing usual depression care with care manager intervention suggested better clinical outcomes when these supportive activities were provided in a more formal way using a care management approach [28]. This care management by an office nurse focused on educating patients, monitoring response to treatment in person and by telephone, and notifying the physician when treatment adjustments were needed [28]. Two caveats are that the study addressed adult depression, not late-life depression, and that better outcomes were observed among patients who had psychologic symptoms rather than physical symptoms.

After the primary care provider and office staff have implemented strategies to prevent suicide, initiated education, and provided basic support, psychotherapy and pharmacotherapy should be considered. Many types of psychotherapy and a number of classes of antidepressants are available and are discussed briefly.

A detailed description of the various psychotherapeutic approaches is beyond the scope of this article, but specific psychotherapeutic approaches can be effective alone or in combination with antidepressant drugs [1,7]. The primary care provider's knowledge about the approaches and skills of local mental health professionals and the ability to make timely referrals may be just as important in treatment as knowledge of antidepressant drugs. In general, interpersonal therapy, a variant of cognitive-behavioral therapy, is more effective than insight-oriented or psychoanalytic psychotherapy [1]. The interpersonal therapy approach addresses and attempts to correct the negative thinking that contributes to sustaining the depressed state and focuses especially on the negative thinking involved in interpersonal interactions [1]. Another approach, brief dynamic therapy, is also efficacious in the treatment of late-life depression [29]. Brief dynamic therapy uses the collaborative aspects of the patient–therapist alliance to problem solve rather than the transference that characterizes classic dynamic therapy.

A comprehensive review and a discussion of pharmacotherapy for depressive disorders are also beyond the scope of this article, but a few basic principles are presented. As is true for the psychotherapeutic approaches just described, drug therapy has been shown to improve outcomes for persons with late-life depression. All of the drugs approved by the Food and Drug Administration for the treatment of depression can be used in the older adult, but drug selection for the individual patient often depends on one or more of the following factors: (1) coexisting medical and neuropsychiatric conditions and concomitant drug therapy for those conditions, (2) expected side-effect profile of the given antidepressant, (3) previous response to antidepressants if known, and (4) the cost of the given antidepressant or its availability based on limitations imposed by a formulary or by a prior authorization program. Before starting an antidepressant, findings from the history and physical examination, including blood pressure readings in the supine and standing positions, should be reviewed. Liver and renal studies should be reviewed because most antidepressants are metabolized in the liver and excreted in the urine. Electrocardiographic findings of left bundle branch block, bifascicular block, second-degree heart block, or QT prolongation or the presence of atrial fibrillation should prompt consideration of a cardiology consultation before initiating antidepressant therapy.

The available classes of antidepressants are shown in Table 1 [1]. Table 1 is not all-inclusive but provides a framework for considering risks and benefits of the various classes of antidepressants and of some of the drugs within each class. The biochemical underpinnings of the treatment of major depression involve manipulating multiple neurotransmitters and their receptors but focus on norepinephrine and 5-hydroxytryptamine. An

Table 1
Available classes of antidepressants

Drug	Dose/d (initial maintenance) (mg)	Therapeutic serum level (ng/dL)	Relative sedation	Relative anticholinergic	Postural hypotension
Heterocyclics					
Doxepin	25–100	>100	++++	++++	++++
Nortriptyline	10–75	50–150	+++	+++	+++
Desipramine	25–125	>125	++	++	+++
Trazodone	50–300	NA	++++	+	+++
Nefazodone	100–600	NA	+++	+	+
SSRIs					
Fluoxetine	5–20	NA	+	+	+
Sertraline	25–100	NA	+	+	+
Paroxetine	10–20	NA	+	++	+
Citalopram	20–40	NA	+	+	+
Others					
Venlafaxine (S/NRI)	25–75	NA	+	+	+
Mirtazapine	15–45	NA	+++	+	+
Bupropion	75–300	NA	+	+	+
MAO inhibitors					
Phenelzine	15–45	>80% inhibition of MAO	+	++	+++
Mood stabilizers					
Lithium carbonate	150–600	0.4–0.7 mmol/L	++	0	0
Valproic acid	250–1250	50–100 ng/mL	++	0	0
Stimulants					
Methylphenidate	5–30	NA	0	0	?

Abbreviations: MAO, monoamine oxidase; NA, not applicable; S/NRI, serotonin/norepinephrine reuptake inhibitor; SSRI, selective serotonin reuptake inhibitor; four plus signs, strong; three plus signs, moderate; two plus signs, weak; one plus sign, negligible; zero, none; question mark, uncertain.

Data from Koenig HG, Blazer DG. Depression, anxiety, and other mood disorders. In: Cassel CK, Leipzig RM, Cohen HJ, et al, editors. Geriatric medicine: an evidence based approach. 4th edition. New York: Springer-Verlag; 2003. p. 1168, 1171.

increase in 5-hydroxytryptamine transmission and probably an increase in norepinephrine transmission appear to be necessary for successful treatment of major depression [30]. Tricyclic antidepressants (TCAs), such as nortriptyline and desipramine, affect uptake of norepinephrine and 5-hydroxytryptamine or of norepinephrine alone, whereas selective serotonin reuptake inhibitors (SSRIs) act specifically to block 5-hydroxytryptamine uptake with little or no effect on norepinephrine [30]. Duloxetine (not listed in Table 1) and venlafaxine affect serotonin and norepinephrine neurotransmission [1,31].

Although TCAs and SSRIs are equally effective in the treatment of depression, SSRIs are now used more widely than TCAs or any other class of antidepressants [1,7]. The unwanted effects of TCAs include postural hypotension, anticholinergic symptoms, and cardiac conduction problems [1]. These side effects are associated more often with the tertiary-amine TCAs such as amitriptyline than with the secondary-amine TCAs such as nortriptyline and desipramine, which are listed in Table 1. The tertiary-amine TCAs have no place in the treatment of depression in the older adult. Secondary-amine TCAs are potentially useful in severe depression with melancholic symptoms [1]. Although SSRIs are prescribed frequently for late-life depression, they are not without side effects. Common side effects of SSRIs include gastrointestinal symptoms, weight loss, tremor, disequilibrium, insomnia, and excessive stimulation and agitation [1]. In addition, specific SSRIs interfere with various components of the P-450 system, thus altering the metabolism of a number of drugs, including warfarin, cimetidine, and the quinolone antibiotics among others [1]. SSRIs also may be associated with inappropriate secretion of vasopressin, especially among the very old [1].

Venlafaxine, mirtazapine, and bupropion are not SSRIs or TCAs but each is effective in treating late-life depression. As noted earlier, venlafaxine inhibits reuptake of norepinephrine and serotonin. It has been associated with worsening of hypertension; therefore, blood pressure should be monitored closely when venlafaxine is prescribed [1]. Mirtazapine is sedating, especially at a dose of 15 mg daily, and can be useful if insomnia is a prominent symptom [1]. Mirtazapine is also said to be useful in treating depression in the older patient who has anorexia or weight loss [32,33]. Bupropion may be useful in patients who have psychomotor retardation or in those who are poorly motivated, fatigued, or frail and in patients who are at risk for falls [1]. Higher doses of bupropion have been associated with tremor, gastrointestinal side effects, and visual hallucinations; bupropion should not be used if there is a history of seizures [1].

Trazodone has been used to treat agitated depression due to its sedating effect. It does not have significant anticholinergic effects but is associated with postural hypotension and priapism [1].

Patients who have late-life depression and are medically ill, anorexic, or apathetic are potential candidates for low-dose methylphenidate [1]. In a study published almost 20 years ago, three fourths of medical and surgical patients who had depression showed improvement after being treated with dextroamphetamine or methylphenidate [34]. A more recent study described the usefulness of methylphenidate augmentation of citalopram in 10 elderly patients who had a mean age of 79.8 years [35].

Because most clinical trials of antidepressant treatments are conducted in younger patients, consensus guidelines by expert panels continue to be useful in our approach to late-life depression. The findings of a well-conceived and meticulously conducted consensus process generated the recommendations for mild and severe unipolar nonpsychotic major depression depicted in Table 2 [36].

Monitoring response to treatment

How should outcomes be monitored in the primary care office setting? Major depression is a serious condition in older adults, and under the best of circumstances, response to therapy may take 4 to 6 weeks. The care management approach previously described suggests that frequent contact by telephone or in person improves outcomes [28]. Office–patient inter-actions in the first 1 to 2 weeks should focus on further educational efforts and identifying and addressing side effects. Over the next 4 to 6 weeks, interactions should assess the extent to which symptoms resolve and the extent to which function and quality of life improve. Each component of the multifaceted intervention should be scrutinized, including the supportive activities and psychotherapeutic approaches employed and the effectiveness of the selected antidepressant. If improvement is not seen at the optimal dose of the initial antidepressant, then the primary care provider should review the process by which the diagnosis was reached and choose another class of antidepressants or refer to psychiatry.

How long should treatment be continued if the person with late-life depression responds to treatment? If the older person is in remission after a single lifetime episode of severe unipolar nonpsychotic depression, then most experts recommend discontinuing treatment after 1 year [36]. With two episodes, there is less agreement, with 10% of the experts recommending 1 year of therapy, 39% recommending 2 years, 14% recommending 3 years, and 37% recommending longer than 3 years [36]. For patients who have had three episodes, essentially 100% of the experts would treat for more than 3 years [36].

Table 2
Consensus recommendations about treatment strategies and medication selection

Treatment strategies	Mild depression		Severe depression	
	Preferred	Alternate	Preferred	Alternate
Overall initial treatment strategies	Antidepressant medication plus psychotherapy	Antidepressant medication alone Psychotherapy alone	Antidepressant medication plus psychotherapy[a] Antidepressant medication alone	Electroconvulsive therapy
Choice of antidepressants	SSRIs[a] Venlafaxine XR	Bupropion Mirtazapine	SSRIs[a] Venlafaxine XR	TCAs Mirtazapine Bupropion

XR, extended release.
[a] Treatment of choice.
Data from Alexopoulos GS, Katz IR, Reynolds CF, et al. The expert opinion guideline series: pharmacotherapy of depressive disorders in older patients. Postgrad Med Special Rep 2001;Oct:24.

Summary

Older adults who visit the primary care physician's office often exhibit depressive symptoms. The challenge for the physician and other office staff is to determine what these symptoms mean: Loneliness? Fear? Grief? A consequence of a coexisting medical condition? A DSM depressive disorder? Or something else?

Addressing ambiguous symptoms that may represent a depressive disorder may be difficult in the busy office setting. The findings of one recent study suggest that it is not lack of knowledge that impedes the recognition of depression but rather the conditions under which clinical decision making occurs [37]. The process of ruling out medical diagnoses and opening the door to consider a mental health diagnosis can be time-consuming and circuitous, especially if the clinician is not already familiar with the patient or if the clinician who is familiar with the patient perceives insufficient time to deal with the issues raised by opening the door [37]. The fundamental challenge for the primary care clinician as aging baby boomers inundate the health care system is to restructure office practice to recognize, assess, and manage geriatric syndromes including depression. The underlying principle for successful restructuring is acknowledging that these syndromes have multiple causes requiring multifaceted interventions. Operationally, doing simple things consistently and well may have significant impact. By consistently recognizing biologic and psychosocial risk factors for depression, by taking a careful history (including the two-question screen [25]), and by conducting a thorough physical examination, the office-based clinician will generally have a strong clinical hunch about the presence or absence of a depressive disorder and any comorbid medical and neuropsychiatric conditions. Armed with this information, additional laboratory and brain imaging studies and subsequent management strategies are straightforward.

References

[1] Koenig HG, Blazer DG. Depression, anxiety, and other mood disorders. In: Cassel CK, Leipzig RM, Cohen HJ, et al, editors. Geriatric medicine: an evidence-based approach. 4th edition. New York: Springer-Verlag; 2003. p. 1163–83.

[2] American Psychological Association. Diagnostic and statistical manual of mental disorders. 4th edition. Washington, DC: American Psychological Association; 1994.

[3] Beekman AT, Geerlings SW, Deeg DJ, et al. The natural history of late-life depression: a 6-year prospective study in the community. Arch Gen Psychiatry 2002;59(7):605–11.

[4] Hybels CF, Blazer DG. Epidemiology of late-life mental disorders. Clin Geriatr Med 2003; 19(4):663–96.

[5] Kaufman SR, Shim JK, Russ AJ. Revisiting the biomedicalization of aging: clinical trends and ethical challenges. Gerontologist 2004;44(6):731–8.

[6] Krishnan KR, Taylor WD, McQuoid DR, et al. Clinical characteristics of magnetic resonance imaging-defined subcortical ischemic depression. Biol Psychiatry 2004;55(4): 390–7.

[7] Blazer DG. Depression in late life: review and commentary. J Gerontol A Biol Sci Med Sci 2003;58(3):249–65.

[8] MacDonald AJD. Do general practitioners miss depression in elderly patients? BMJ 1986; 292:1365–7.

[9] Fyffe DC, Sirey JA, Heo M, et al. Late-life depression among black and white elderly homecare patients. Am J Geriatr Psychiatry 2004;12(5):531–5.

[10] Parmelee P, Katz I, Lawton M. Depression among institutionalized aged: assessment and prevalence estimation. J Gerontol Med Sci 1989;44:M22–9.

[11] Bruce ML. Psychosocial risk factors for depressive disorders in late life. Biol Psychiatry 2002; 52(3):175–84.

[12] Tiemeier H. Biological risk factors for late life depression. Eur J Epidemiol 2003;18(8): 745–50.

[13] Charlson M, Peterson JC. Medical comorbidity and late-life depression: what is known and what are unmet needs? Biol Psychiatry 2002;52(3):226–35.

[14] Tupler LA, Krishnan KR, MacDonald WM, et al. Anatomic location and laterality of MRI intensities in late-life depression. J Psychosom Res 2002;53(2):665–76.

[15] Mast BT, Neufield S, MacNeill SE, et al. Longitudinal support for the relationship between vascular risk factors and late-life depressive symptoms. Am J Geriatr Psychiatry 2004;12(1): 93–101.

[16] Krishnan MS, Mast BT, Ficker LJ, et al. The effects of pre-existing depression on cerebrovascular health outcomes in geriatric continuing care. J Gerontol Med Sci, in press.

[17] Krishnan KR. Biological risk factors in late life depression. Biol Psychiatry 2002;52(3): 185–92.

[18] Williams JR. Depression as mediator between spousal bereavement and mortality from cardiovascular disease: appreciating and managing the adverse health consequences of depression in an elderly surviving spouse. Sout Med J 2005;98(1):90–5.

[19] Schulz R, Beach SR, Lind B, et al. Involvement in caregiving and adjustment to death of a spouse: findings from the caregiver health effects study. JAMA 2001;285(24): 3123–9.

[20] US Preventive Services Task Force. Screening: depression. Available at: http://www.ahrq. gov/clinic/uspsdepr.htm. Accessed March 8, 2005.

[21] Lyness JM, Noel TK, Cox C, et al. Screening for depression in elderly primary care patients. A comparison of the CES-D and the GDS. Arch Intern Med 1997;157(4):449–54.

[22] Klinkman MS, Coyne JC, Gallo S, et al. Can case-finding instruments be used to improve physician detection of depression in primary case? Arch Fam Med 1997;6(6):567–73.

[23] Flocke SA, Frank SH, Wenger DA. Addressing multiple problems in the family practice office visit. J Fam Pract 2001;50:211–6.

[24] Ebell MH. Routine screening for depression. Alcohol problems, and domestic violence. Am Fam Physician 2004;69(10):2421–2.

[25] Whooley MA, Avins AL, Miranda J, et al. Case-finding instruments for depression. Two questions are as good as many. J Gen Intern Med 1997;12:439–45.

[26] Williams R, Vinson DC. Validation of a single screening question for problem drinking. J Fam Pract 2001;50:307–12.

[27] Norman MA, Whooley ME, Kewchang L. Depression and other mental health issues. In: Landefeld CS, Palmer RM, Johnson MA, et al, editors. Current geriatric diagnosis and treatment. New York: Lange Medical Books/McGraw-Hill; 2004. p. 100–13.

[28] Dickinson LM, Rost K, Nutting PA, et al. RCT of a care manager intervention for major depression in primary care: 2-year costs for patients with physical vs. psychological complaints. Ann Fam Med 2005;3:15–22.

[29] Thompson LW, Gallagher D, Breckenridge JS. Comparative effectiveness of psychotherapies for depressed elders. J Consult Clin Psychol 1987;55:385–90.

[30] Gareri P, De Fazio P, De Sarro G. Neuropharmacology of depression in aging and age-related diseases. Ageing Res Rev 2002;1(1):113–34.

[31] Lilly Research Laboratories. Cymbalta package insert. Available at: http://pi.lilly.com/us/cymbalta-pi.pdf. Accessed March 13, 2005.

[32] Morley JE. Orexigenic and anabolic agents. Clin Geriatr Med 2002;18(4):853–66.

[33] Raji MA, Brady SR. Mirtazapine for treatment of depression and comorbidities in Alzheimer disease. Ann Pharmacother 2001;35(9):1024–7.

[34] Woods SW, Tesar GE, Murray GB, et al. Psychostimulant treatment of depressive disorders secondary to medical illness. J Clin Psychiatry 1986;47(1):12–5.

[35] Lavretsky H, Kumar A. Methylphenidate augmentation of citalopram in elderly depressed patients. Am J Geriatr Psychiatry 2001;9(3):298–303.

[36] Alexopoulos GS, Katz IR, Reynolds CF, et al. The expert opinion guideline series: pharmacotherapy of depressive disorders in older patients. Postgrad Med Special Rep 2001; Oct:1–88.

[37] Baik SY, Bowers BJ, Oakley LD, Susman JL. The recognition of depression: the primary care clinician's perspective. Ann Fam Med 2005;3:31–7.

ELSEVIER
SAUNDERS

Prim Care Clin Office Pract
32 (2005) 793–810

PRIMARY CARE:
CLINICS IN
OFFICE PRACTICE

The Primary Care Physician's Role in Nursing Facility Care

Seki A. Balogun, MD*, Jonathan Evans, MD, MPH

*Division of General Medicine, Geriatrics, and Palliative Care,
Department of Internal Medicine, University of Virginia Health System,
P.O. Box 800901, Charlottesville, VA 22908-0506, USA*

The purpose of this article is to help physicians who care for nursing facility residents understand their role as care providers in the nursing facility setting and to provide information of use to physicians in carrying out their role. In addition, the nursing facility environment and a number of other factors important to the care of older patients in nursing facilities are discussed to demonstrate the context within which the primary care physician's role must fit. The care of a patient focuses primarily on the individual's medical condition regardless of the care setting but is dependent on the setting to a certain extent. A physician caring for nursing facility residents must understand the care environment to provide the highest quality of care in that setting. Every physician should know what he or she can reasonably expect from the facility and what patients, families, facility staff, regulators, and payors can expect of the physician.

Nursing facilities are highly regulated, and several federal regulations applicable to nursing facilities specifically deal with physician conduct, such as the minimum frequency of physician visits, drug prescribing, physical restraint use, care plan development and oversight, interaction with consultant pharmacists, and the timeliness of orders for care. Consequently, physicians caring for nursing facility residents must be familiar with applicable regulations and must have some understanding of systems of care delivery in the nursing facility.

The need for caring, competent, and committed physicians in long-term care is great and expected to increase. As the population ages and as acute care hospital length-of-stay patterns continue to shorten, the number of Americans requiring nursing facility placement following acute care

* Corresponding author.
E-mail address: sab2s@virginia.edu (S.A. Balogun).

0095-4543/05/$ - see front matter © 2005 Elsevier Inc. All rights reserved.
doi:10.1016/j.pop.2005.06.010   *primarycare.theclinics.com*

hospitalization will continue to rise. As a result, physicians in virtually every specialty who provide hospital care must have at least a basic working knowledge of nursing facility care to safely and appropriately transfer patients from the acute care hospital to the nursing facility. As more and more patients require at least short-term nursing facility care, primary care physicians in particular will increasingly be called on to serve as attending physicians for an increasing number of medically complex residents of nursing facilities [1]. Based on current trends, it is estimated that most Americans aged 65 years and older will reside in a nursing home at some point in their lifetime for short-term rehabilitation or long-term care [2,3]. As the elderly population increases over the next several decades, long-term care facilities may become major sites where primary care physician services are needed.

Historical background and context

The concept of nursing homes dates at least as far back as twelfth-century Greece, where the elderly were cared for in special, highly esteemed infirmaries called "gerocomeia" that were run mostly in or near monasteries [4]. In Europe, special care units for the chronically ill elderly were developed between 1900 and 1950 in response to the problematic status of these patients in the workhouses and general hospitals [5]. In the United States, nursing homes, as we know them today, were developed in the early 1900s. Most residents were the chronically ill or disabled. Even then, most assistance to the elderly poor population came from the county-run poorhouses.

State licensure programs were developed in the 1920s, but standards and oversight were minimal and focused primarily on building and safety codes [6].

Following passage of the Social Security Act in the mid-1900s, poor-houses (not entitled to Social Security funds) gave way to private nursing homes that were allowed to receive such funds. Often, these facilities were converted farmhouses, mansions, or motels with poor safety features and wide variations in care. Many were not equipped to care for frail or ill elderly residents and provided only a room and meals. These facilities were run mainly by nurses, with most of the care being custodial in nature [6].

A post-World War II building boom saw the development of nursing homes that were modeled after hospitals in appearance and that took on a distinctively medical look. Nevertheless, the care that was provided continued to vary widely. Many nursing facilities received payment from Medicaid; however, there were minimal federal standards for the care provided. Following several well-publicized scandals and some tragic accidents, momentum grew for greater governmental oversight, prompting the federal government to commission a study by the Institute of Medicine. The Institute of Medicine report served as a blueprint for sweeping governmental reform soon afterward. In 1987, the Nursing Home Reform Act was passed as part of an omnibus spending bill, the Omnibus Budget

Reconciliation act of 1987 since referred to as OBRA '87. The 1980s also saw the introduction of significant changes in Medicare payment to hospitals, with lump-sum payment for hospitalization according to Diagnosis-Related Groups rather than fee-for-service payment based on daily hospital charges. This prospective payment system provided strong financial incentives for shorter hospital stays. As a result, transfers to skilled nursing homes following a qualifying acute care hospital stay rose dramatically, and nursing facility care shifted toward care of sicker and more medically complex patients. It has often been said that the nursing home of today looks like the hospital of yesterday; more precisely, it looks increasingly like the ICU.

Since the 1980s, nursing homes have gradually evolved into facilities that care for the functionally and cognitively impaired, with state regulations to ensure quality of care. By law, all nursing homes now have a medical director who is part of the administrative body of these institutions. The medical director provides oversight of the medical practice and helps with the implementation of facility. Medical care is rendered to residents by attending physicians with or without physician assistants and nurse practitioners. Nursing care is provided by nurses (licensed practical nurses and registered nurses), with certified nursing assistants providing most of the residents' personal care. Occupational therapists, physical therapists, and speech therapists provide rehabilitative therapies. Other members of the health care team in the nursing home include pharmacists, who usually provide consultative services, and other practitioners, who provide in-house consultative services. These consultative services vary across different institutions and often include podiatrists, optometrists, psychiatrists, and psychologists.

The nature of long-term care has changed dramatically over time, with a variety of forces mostly aimed at cost-containment in hospital settings, resulting in a further shift of care away from the acute care hospitals and into nursing facilities. Hospital length-of-stay patterns continue to shrink for virtually every medical condition, creating a tremendous increase in the number and complexity of recently hospitalized patients receiving aggressive posthospital care in nursing facilities. The population of nursing facility residents has thus gotten "sicker," resulting in the need for a stronger presence by physicians in long-term care facilities.

Epidemiology

Reaching old age in the United States has become commonplace. The median age of the population is increasing because of a decline in fertility and a 20-year increase in the average life span during the second half of the twentieth century [7].

According to the 2003 United States population estimates, Americans older than 65 years make up about 14% of the total population. By the year 2020, one in five Americans will be older than 65 years [8].

Forty-three percent of adults older than 65 years will enter a nursing home at some time before they die. Of those who enter nursing homes, 55% will have total lifetime use of at least 1 year and 21% will have total lifetime use of 5 years or more.

Worldwide, the average life span is expected to extend another 10 years by 2050. Chronic diseases, which affect older adults disproportionately, contribute to disability, diminish quality of life, and increase long-term care use and costs [7].

Overview of nursing facilities

At present, there are approximately 1.5 million Americans, most aged 65 years and older, living in 17,000 nursing facilities nationwide [9]. In addition, the number of assisted living facilities, in which at least hundreds of thousands of other older Americans reside, is increasing rapidly.

The demographics of nursing home residents are also rapidly changing, with residents being increasingly more medically complex and frail. With today's elderly population living and staying healthier longer, other options such as assisted living programs and community-based adult day care facilities are used until individual care needs can no longer be met [10]. As such, nursing homes often are the option of last resort, especially in rural areas, where there are fewer assisted living facilities [11].

In general, the assisted living industry has attempted to develop facilities that are physically attractive alternatives to nursing homes for older people requiring some supervision or physical assistance due to impairments attributed to chronic diseases. At the same time, many nursing facilities have attempted to shift their emphasis from the long-term care of patients who have dementia and other chronic conditions to subacute care and rehabilitation for patients' complex medical conditions.

Nursing facilities are often part of a larger private organization, a community or teaching hospital, or a health maintenance organization [12,13]. A large number of nursing homes have an open medical staff policy whereby any physician is allowed to admit and care for patients in the facility. An advantage of this policy is that it allows for continuity of care because the patient's physician can continue to provide medical care across different settings (from the ambulatory outpatient setting to the acute inpatient setting to the long-term care setting).

Some nursing homes have a closed admission system whereby a few physicians, often employed full-time by the facility, provide medical care. The potential advantage in this model is greater physician availability [14].

Types of care in nursing facilities

Traditionally, care in the nursing home differs from care in other settings, in that the goal is not to cure an illness but to allow an individual to achieve and maintain an optimal level of functioning. The care encompasses an array of medical, social, personal, and supportive and specialized housing services needed by individuals who have lost some capacity for self-care because of a chronic illness or disabling condition [15].

Medical care in the nursing home traditionally falls into two main categories: skilled nursing care or rehabilitation and long-term nursing care. More recently, hospice care is being offered in nursing homes.

Skilled nursing care and rehabilitation

Residents requiring skilled nursing care and rehabilitation are typically those discharged from the acute inpatient setting with significant functional deficits and who at times have complex medical illnesses, with the aim to restore sufficient function so that they can return to independent living. These patients often require a high degree of nursing care, which could involve intravenous therapy, extensive wound care, and one or more of the different forms of therapy (physical, occupational, speech). The typical length of stay for these patients in nursing facilities is usually less than 6 months, ranging from a few days to months.

Long-term care

Long-term nursing care residents are those who, due to significant functional, cognitive, or psychosocial issues, require assistance with self-care and other instrumental activities of daily living and can no longer live independently in the community. Many long-term care residents also have poor social support.

Hospice care

Hospice care is increasingly becoming an essential service in nursing facilities. Hospice serves patients who have terminal conditions who typically have less than 6 months to live. Care is usually administered in conjunction with an independent hospice organization or in a hospice unit that maybe part of the nursing facility. The hospice team usually comprises physicians, nurses, social workers, and chaplains—all forming a network of medical, spiritual, and social support for patient and family.

Rules and regulations (the "regulatory environment")

Omnibus Budget Reconciliation Act of 1987

In 1987, federal regulations were enacted governing nursing facilities that accept Medicaid or Medicare payment. These regulations were in response to growing public concern about inconsistent standards, variable nursing facility quality, and a steady increase in federal spending for nursing facility care. These regulations were included in the much larger congressional spending bill, OBRA '87. In response to this federal legislation, each of the 50 states enacted state legislation that is consistent with these federal rules. OBRA '87 had an immediate and profound effect on nursing facility care and the way that nursing facilities are organized and administered. In addition to the regulations themselves, the process created by the federal government and administered by state agencies to evaluate each facility's compliance with these regulations (hence referred to as the "state survey") has had a profound effect on nursing facility culture. These evaluations typically involve yearly unannounced inspections or surveys [16]. Centers for Medicare and Medicaid Services administer the Medicare and Medicaid programs and the regulations for the nursing facilities [17].

According to OBRA '87 regulations, each facility is required to have a physician medical director and must have certain committees (eg, quality assurance and infection control) in place that meet with a minimum frequency (at least quarterly). OBRA '87 regulations further required that nursing facilities must establish their own written policies and procedures covering a wide range of subjects, including everything from emergency evacuation to food preparation and handling to medication administration. Facility staff must notify the resident's family and physician in a timely manner in the event of an acute change in condition. Each facility must obtain the services of a consultant pharmacist whose responsibility it is to review the medications of each resident at least every 30 days and communicate any concerns to the resident's physician and facility administration.

Individual facilities may require physicians to abide by certain policies and procedures before assuming care of the residents in a nursing home, which often involve formal documents stating the obligations of the physicians. Most facilities also require verification of the physician's credentials before privileges are granted. Medical practice in long-term care is the most regulated of the different patient care sites. In addition to OBRA '87 regulations, some nursing homes are voluntarily accredited by the Joint Commission on Accreditation of Health Care Organizations, which is an independent, not-for-profit organization and the nation's predominant standards-setting and accrediting body in health care [18]. Nursing homes are also subject to regulatory oversight by other agencies such as the Occupational Health and Safety Administration, which assures the safety and health of America's workers by setting and enforcing standards to ensure safety and health in the workplace [19], and the Health Insurance Portability and Accountability Act, which helped establish national standards for electronic health care transactions, security, and privacy of health data [20].

To assure compliance with federal regulations, a process of unannounced on-site inspections (occurring at least annually) was developed, along with a process for unannounced inspections in response to specific complaints. These inspections, conducted by investigators from each state's department of health under contract from the federal Centers for Medicare and Medicaid Services, are referred to as the state survey. A team of investigators (the survey team) performs an on-site inspection of the facility that includes direct observation of caregivers, interviews with residents and staff, and a review of medical records and written policies and procedures. The team is required to look for and report any incidents or areas of deficient practice or "deficiencies" (ie, failures to comply with federal or state regulations) and to communicate their findings to the facility. The facility must then submit a formal plan of correction to the health department, which, depending on the scope and severity of the deficiencies cited, may accept the plan of correction as evidence of substantial compliance with those regulations or may require a follow-up investigation (survey) to directly ascertain whether the facility is now in compliance. Severe deficiencies may result in substantial civil penalties including fines, exclusion from participation as health care providers in Medicaid and Medicare programs, and revocation of license.

Attending physician roles in long-term care

The primary care physician plays a critical role in promoting, maintaining, and restoring health for individual patients. For ambulatory patients living independently in the community, this role is primarily performed during patients' visits to the physician's office. For residents of nursing facilities, the attending physician has an even more expanded role. The physician is specifically charged with helping to develop a comprehensive care plan for each patient's care, with care provided by an interdisciplinary team. The physician must give written orders for care and oversee the care provided by all of the interdisciplinary care team members at the facility. For patients receiving skilled care services, the physician must certify the need for skilled care at the time of admission and periodically recertify the need for ongoing skilled care.

Physician visits

Over the last century, the physician's office has been the principal site for ambulatory care delivery in the United States. In general, the layout, staffing, and stocking of equipment and supplies in the physician's office are designed to promote efficiency in care delivery, convenience for the physician, and a measure of convenience for patients. The office also represents a substantial investment in equipment and overhead expense for the practitioner. Thus, there are strong financial pressures and incentives to keep office-based physicians in the clinic rather than seeing patients off-site. Nevertheless, a significant number of older patients, particularly those with physical or cognitive impairment may find it difficult or impossible to make and keep an office appointment without the assistance of others (particularly family members) in seeking care, providing or arranging transportation, and accompanying them to the office appointment. This is often inconvenient, if not expensive, for family members or other caregivers, although the visit itself may be worth it for many.

Nursing facility residents may be seen in physicians' offices; however, unless they are being seen for a procedure that is best performed in a clinic setting, there are several important reasons, in addition to those already noted, that make it preferable for physicians to visit their nursing home patients at the facility (Table 1).

The quality of the medical history may be enhanced by visiting the patient at the facility rather than the office, particularly for cognitively impaired patients. History provided by facility staff is often invaluable. In addition, the ability to review the nursing home chart in its entirety cannot be underestimated. A history obtained in the office may be unreliable or incomplete.

Assessment of function and well-being is often best done by observing patients in their environment and by observing their interactions with staff and other residents. Repeated observation over time also gives insight into patients' habits and may offer additional clues to the development of illness when routines change or function declines.

Visiting patients at the facility provides greater opportunity for communication between the physician and facility staff, and generally results in better communication overall. Having an opportunity to interact with the staff who provide direct care to patients is invaluable and can improve staff and patient morale.

Seeing nursing facility residents at the facility is often more efficient than seeing them in the office and can potentially cut down on the number of

Table 1
Advantages of nursing facility patient visits

Variables	Nursing facility patient visit	Office visit
History taking	Can corroborate history with nursing facility staff	May be unreliable and incomplete, especially with cognitively impaired patients
Assessment of function and well-being	Patients can be observed in their usual environment	Difficult to fully assess patients outside their own environment
Care planning and oversight	Easier to collaborate with the nursing staff and other caregivers in facility	May be more difficult
Improved communication with staff and family	Meeting caregivers and staff in nursing home facilitates better communication	May not be practical to meet nursing staff and caregiver in office setting
Efficiency	More efficient: less distractions and less time constraints	May be more distractions

office distractions such as phone calls and faxes that may interfere with patient flow.

Although it may not always be convenient for the physician, the convenience afforded to patients, families, and the facility caregivers is great. Family members must often take time away from work to bring their loved one to the office. If facility staff members are needed to transport or accompany residents to a doctor's office visit, fewer staff are available to provide care to the other residents of the facility. Moreover, patients and families may sometimes incur additional transportation costs to get an immobile nursing facility resident to the office.

Attending physicians must evaluate and treat nursing facility residents as often as medically necessary. Irrespective of the patient's health status at the time of the visit and even without a specific request from the patient or his or her family, federal and state regulations require that the attending physician provide physician visits with a certain minimum frequency to oversee and certify the appropriateness of nursing facility care and renew written orders for care. Thus, these visits are often referred to as "recertification visits" or "periodic visits" by many physicians. Patients admitted to the nursing facility must have to their treatment orders approved on admission and should be seen by a physician within 48 to 72 hours. Existing literature suggests that the quality of care in various patient care settings including nursing homes is directly related to the degree of physician involvement [21].

The minimum frequency of recertification visits varies by payor source and by state law. For example, Medicare requires that Medicare Part A recipients residing in nursing facilities and receiving skilled care under Medicare Part A must be seen by a physician at least once every 30 days for the first 90 days and at least once every 60 days thereafter. Medicaid requires that recipients residing in nursing facilities be seen by a physician at least once every 60 days. State laws may also set a minimum frequency for physician visits to long-term care facility residents but can never be less stringent than Medicare and Medicaid regulations. Orders for care must also be renewed every 30 or 60 days.

Medicare or Medicaid does not limit the frequency with which patients in nursing facilities must be seen. How often a nursing facility resident is seen by his or her physician in between periodic visits is based on medical necessity. It is not unusual for ill patients to be seen at least weekly over extended periods of time or for sick patients and patients who have complex problems recently transferred from the acute care hospital to require daily visits for a short period of time.

Periodic physician visits allow an opportunity for medical assessment and provide an opportunity to review the comprehensive care plan and orders for care. These visits are an opportunity to (1) discontinue medications or treatments that are no longer necessary, (2) review the documentation of other members of the interdisciplinary care team in the patient's chart, (3) review the federally mandated Minimum Data Set and other resident assessments,

(4) discuss the patient's condition and care with family members and nursing facility staff, (5) decide on the appropriateness and frequency of particular preventive health and screening interventions for individual patients, and (6) assess the appropriateness and results of laboratory and diagnostic tests as necessary. Other issues that may at times be relevant components of periodic visits are (1) evaluation of urinary catheters and other devices to determine the appropriateness of ongoing use; (2) evaluation of recurrent falls; (3) evaluation, treatment, and monitoring of pressure sores; and (4) assessment of the appropriateness of restraint use.

Physician availability

Physicians are required to be available or to have a designated backup physician available by way of phone or pager 24 hours a day, 7 days a week. It is important for attending physicians to understand the nursing facility environment and culture and to realize that failures on the part of attending physicians (such as failing to see patients in a timely manner, failing to document an appropriate indication for the use of certain medications, or failing to evaluate certain conditions such as unexplained weight loss) may result in sanctions against the facility itself, although not necessarily against the physician. Nursing facilities can be punished for any of their own failings and for what attending physicians do or do not do.

Understanding the regulatory environment is important to understanding why nursing facilities operate the way they do and why some facilities and staff may at times appear rule bound and fearful. Attending physicians must understand, for example, that the many phone calls, faxes, and mailed communications generated by the facility, including orders for care that require prompt signature, are generally in direct response to regulations requiring physician notification and response.

Care plan development and oversight

Fragmentation of care across multiple settings and multiple providers makes care coordination increasingly important. Hospitalized patients are discharged to nursing homes "sicker and quicker," creating new challenges for nursing facilities.

In the nursing facility, physicians often provide oversight for the medical care of patients and work with other members of the interdisciplinary team to help each resident achieve the highest practicable level of physical, mental, and psychosocial well-being.

Communication with staff and families

It is important for physicians to communicate with residents' families and include them in the decision-making process with regard to care of their loved ones. Family involvement and family-oriented practices are invaluable in the nursing home. They often promote a great relationship between the staff, the resident, and the resident's family, and give the family and resident a sense of control over the resident's care [22,23].

Medication prescribing

Federal regulations directly affect physician prescribing practices in the nursing facility. Psychotropic medications, for example, can only be administered to treat specific neuropsychiatric conditions. Dementia with agitation or wandering is explicitly listed as inadequate justification for psychotropic drug use. Physicians prescribing psychotropic drugs must provide written justification in the progress notes for their use and make gradual dose reductions in an attempt to discontinue drug use or explain in the medical record why doing so would be harmful. The federal government has also published guidelines for drug dosages in the elderly to assist regulators during their inspections of the facility.

Each resident's drug regimen must be free from "unnecessary drugs." Federal regulations define an unnecessary drug as any drug used in one or more of the following situations: (1) excessive dose or duration (includes duplicate therapy), (2) without adequate monitoring, (3) without adequate indications for its use, or (4) in the presence of adverse consequences.

Physical and chemical restraints

Nursing facility residents have the right to be free from unnecessary physical or chemical restraints. A chemical restraint is defined as a drug used for discipline or convenience to decrease disruptive behavior, without attempting nonpharmacologic alternatives first.

A sedating medication used for purposes other than treatment of medical illness or prescribed in an inappropriate or as-needed manner is also considered a chemical restraint.

Physical restraints may only be used to treat a patient's underlying medical condition and only after other, less-restrictive alternatives have failed. Restraints are defined as virtually anything that restricts a resident's mobility. This includes seat belts, "lap buddies," "merry walkers," and full-length bed rails. Because restraints have not been shown definitively to prevent injury and because of several known complications of their use, physical restraint use should perhaps be thought of as a "stop gap" measure for temporary use in response to urgent situations while the care plan is being revised in response to a change in the resident's condition.

Ethical and legal roles

Physicians in the nursing home are bound by the same principles of medical ethics that are relevant in any area of medical practice. Physicians should also help facilities maintain regulatory compliance and ensure that services provided and ordered are consistent with current standards of medical practice. The nursing facility environment, however, is unique in a number of important ways. Legally, the facility is the patient's "home." Nursing facility residents may be eligible for certain home care services under Medicare, such as hospice benefits, and have additional rights and protections as tenants. The same strict isolation precautions used in hospitals may not be appropriate or necessary in a patient's home, for example, and may therefore not be appropriate in a nursing facility.

Federal regulations grant nursing facility residents specific "resident rights" such as the right to privacy, the right to achieve and maintain the highest level of physical, mental, and psychosocial well-being, the right to be free from unnecessary drugs and physical and chemical restraints. Primary care physicians must be aware of and honor residents' rights. Residents have the right to do well. Consequently, when patients experience a decline in functional status or overall health and well-being, physicians are asked to perform an assessment and to provide appropriate documentation indicating the nature of the problem, what steps are being taken to address it, and expectations for recovery or further decline. Residents in the nursing facility have the right to choose their attending physician, but nursing homes can require that the selected physician fulfills necessary requirements for privileging in the facility.

Residents (or their designated party) also have the right to be fully informed of their treatment plan in a language they understand and be allowed to make decisions regarding their treatment, care plan, and advance directives. In addition, residents have the right to refuse treatment. The physician can guide them in making these decisions, but the residents must be allowed to make their own choices, which must be respected so long as they are consistent with accepted standards of medical care.

Partly as a result of the regulatory environment and a desire to assign responsibility, physicians are often asked to give written orders for things that might not otherwise be thought of as medical care. For example, a patient's ingestion of alcoholic beverages typically requires a physician's order stating the amount and frequency. An order may also be required to allow the resident to leave the facility (their own home) for various reasons. Thus, various aspects of daily life have become "medicalized" in nursing facilities. Primary care physicians should understand the importance that many residents place on personal freedom and even simple choices, particularly when they have little control over many other aspects of their daily lives.

Administrative roles

Physicians with a strong interest in nursing facility care often assume the role of medical director and take on additional responsibilities of assuring the overall quality of care provided to all residents of the facility. Federal regulations require that all nursing home facilities have a physician medical director. The role of the medical director often involves developing and revising policies and standards for patient care, infection control, quality assurance, communicating with other physicians in the facility about policies and standards of care, discussing specific patient problems, assisting in the in-service training of nursing home staff, helping to ensure that emergency care is available, participating in comprehensive care planning, and helping to identify and correct problems in quality of care (Table 2). These responsibilities are often a "part-time" activity because most medical directors also serve as attending physicians for individual facility residents and typically have other responsibilities for patients outside of the facility. Consequently, many medical directors devote less than 4 hours per month solely to medical director activities [24]. Nevertheless, as far as federal and state regulations are concerned, the medical director's responsibility is not in any way diminished if the time spent at the facility is limited.

The amount of interaction between the medical director and the primary care physicians in a facility varies widely. Primary care physicians should be aware that the medical director is responsible for assuring the timeliness of physician visits, the appropriateness of treatment orders, and physician documentation in the medical record. Consequently, medical directors may be called on to perform recertification visits, write orders, or to intervene in emergencies for patients other than their own when necessary.

Primary care physicians who are not medical directors may from time to time also be asked to participate in various administrative activities within the facility, such as participation on the quality assurance committee. There usually is some opportunity for interested physicians to become more

Table 2
Physician roles in nursing homes

Physician roles	Specific duties
Clinical	Resident assessment
	Care plan development and oversight
	Discharge and transfer
	Communication with staff and family
Ethical and legal	Respect residents rights
	Provide clinical care without discrimination
	Aid facilities in maintaining regulatory compliance
Administrative (Medical director)	Participate in administrative decision making
	Help recommend and implement policies and procedures in facility
	Participate in staff educational activities
	Help ensure standard medical care and coordinate physician services
	Help in promoting safety and health of staff

involved to gain a better understanding of care delivery in the facility and of the regulatory environment. Motivated individuals can always make a difference.

Interaction with members of an interdisciplinary team

Long-term care often involves many disciplines: nurses, certified nursing assistants, physical therapists, occupational therapists, speech therapists, dietitians, administrative staff, and numerous consultants such as pharmacists, podiatrists, psychologists, and optometrists. The primary care physician must work as a member of this team to ensure optimal patient care and must foster good communication with other members of the team because this is essential for care planning. In addition, the physician should be aware of the roles and responsibilities of all the other team members involved in the patient's care.

Nurses are an integral part of the team. They administer medications and provide skilled nursing care, which includes wound care, urinary catheter care, intravenous fluids or medications, and phlebotomy for blood laboratory tests. They often function as the attending physician's "eyes and ears," performing assessments and communicating changes in condition and unusual incidents or accidents to the physician. Nurses are charged with the responsibility of directly executing the physicians' orders. These orders are often communicated over the telephone. As such, the importance of adequate communication between physicians and nurses cannot be overemphasized. Some facilities assign specific roles to particular nurses. For example, a facility may employ a wound care nurse whose primary responsibility is to perform wound assessments and treatments on all of the residents rather than on those on a particular wing or floor of the building. A close working relationship with such specialist nurses is often critical for optimal care.

Certified nursing assistants are the front-line caregivers in nursing facilities and represent the largest proportion of facility employees. They are usually responsible for the direct personal day-to-day care of the residents and generally have much more direct patient contact than nurses. Nursing assistants perform a very important function because most nursing home residents require assistance with some aspect of self-care and a large percentage are totally dependent on others for all basic activities of daily living including toileting, feeding, bathing, and dressing. Although not specifically trained to perform patient assessments, their frequent interaction with facility residents makes nursing assistants an invaluable source of information for physicians, particularly when patients have impaired communication ability.

The consultant pharmacist, in accordance with federal regulations, reviews the medications of each nursing facility resident at least monthly and then communicates his or her findings or concerns to the attending physician. This communication between the pharmacist and physician may be verbal; however, most often, written communication is faxed or mailed to the physician for review, response, and signature. Prompt physician response is necessary for patient safety and to help the facility maintain compliance with federal and state regulations.

Frequent, direct communication between physician and pharmacist can be invaluable and is therefore strongly encouraged. The consultant pharmacist is an available resource for attending physicians when making prescribing decisions, including the choice of medication and medication dose. Residents of nursing facilities have the federally protected right to be free from unnecessary drugs and chemical restraints. In addition, the use of antipsychotic and certain other psychoactive medications in nursing facilities is regulated and a frequent source of scrutiny by state surveyors and others as a quality-of-care indicator. The total number of medications prescribed per resident, another quality-of-care indicator, is also scrutinized by regulators. The risk of significant drug–drug interactions and adverse drug events increases with the number of medications prescribed. Monthly medication review by consultant pharmacists serves as an important quality assurance step in identifying potential drug–drug and drug–disease interactions, in identifying medications whose indication is not clearly documented in the medical record, and in reducing overall medication costs.

Other consultants such as podiatrists, psychologists, and optometrists provide services in their area of specialty in the nursing home facility, usually in response to direct referral from the primary care physician. These consultants typically are not facility employees but usually have a written agreement with the facility. Their visits vary widely and are dependent on the needs of the residents. Communication between these consultants and the physician is invaluable to ensure that the residents' needs are adequately addressed. It should be noted that most nursing facilities accept orders for care only from the patient's attending physician. Consequently, attending physicians may routinely be asked to review and verify recommendations made by consultants before those recommendations can be implemented.

Documentation and coding

Primary care physicians should provide adequate documentation in the patient's medical record, as with any other patient care setting. This documentation serves as an important form of communication to other health care providers, payors, and regulators and, at times, is the only form of communication that payors and regulators routinely rely on in assessing the adequacy and appropriateness of care and the appropriate level of reimbursement for care. In addition, documentation in the form of a "billing code" is used to communicate to regulators and payors the nature and scope of physician services provided during a particular visit. The specific documentation requirements vary depending on the type of visit and billing code used.

Table 3
Documentation and billing

Resident assessments	Code	Requirements
Comprehensive nursing facility assessments	99301 Annual assessment of resident not medically complex	Detailed interval history Comprehensive examination Low-complexity medical decision making
	99302 Evaluation of a new or established resident who has experienced a major change in status that is expected to be permanent and has resulted in a nursing facility assessment	Detailed interval history Comprehensive examination Moderate to high-complexity medical decision making New care plan and completion of minimum data set
	99303 Evaluation of a new or established resident at the time of admission or readmission to the facility	Comprehensive history Comprehensive examination Moderate-to high-complexity medical decision making Development of medical care plan
Subsequent nursing facility care	99311 Evaluation of a new or established resident, usually when condition stable, recovering, or improving	Two of three key components: Problem-focused interval history Problem-focused examination Low-complexity medical decision making
	99312 Evaluation of new or established resident, usually when there is inadequate response to therapy or minor complication	Two of three key components: Expanded problem-focused interval history Expanded problem-focused examination Moderate-complexity decision making
	99313 Evaluation of new or established resident, usually when there is a significant complication or new problem	Two of three key components: Detailed interval history Detailed examination Moderate-to high-complexity medical decision making
Discharge planning codes	99315 Nursing facility discharge planning or discharge day management	Total amount of time spent: 30 min or less
	99316 Nursing facility discharge planning or discharge day management	Total amount of time spent: More than 30 min

In general, it is recommended that the reason for the visit and an indication that the health care provider had direct physical contact or interaction with the patient (in form of pertinent medical history, physical findings, laboratory data, assessment, and plan) be documented for each visit. To comply with specific regulatory requirements, attending physicians may be asked by the facility staff or the consultant pharmacist to document the ongoing need for a medication or treatment ordered, the medical decision making involved in choosing a particular medication over others, and the dosage used. Documentation justifying continued use of the medication may also be necessary. Physicians should also document, whenever possible, their expectation of prognosis, especially in cases in which the patient's condition has declined. Physicians may be specifically asked to comment in the chart about conditions such as pressure sores, weight loss, nutritional status, and factors justifying the ongoing provision of skilled care services.

There are eight common evaluation and management codes specific to nursing facility services. These codes are categorized as comprehensive assessments, subsequent care, and discharge planning codes. Although these codes are similar to codes used in office and hospital settings (conceptually and in terms of their required components), a number of key differences exist (Table 3). In addition, certain codes in nursing facilities indicate the patient's overall condition or whether the patient has recently been admitted or readmitted (eg, the nursing facility code 99302 indicates a major change in status). Physicians must at least be aware of the minimum requirements for documentation of each particular code.

Summary

As more care is shifted from the acute care hospital and other sites to nursing facilities, and as the complexity of nursing facility care increases, more is expected of attending physicians. Physicians play an important role in helping patients and their families in this setting and in working with the facility staff in caring for these patients. Structuring visits to address patient and family needs and staff concerns; reviewing resident assessment instruments, care plans, and orders for care; and carefully documenting and coding those visits in such a way as to represent the purpose and complexity of the visit and the patient's clinical circumstances not only helps to improve the overall care provided to the patient but also helps others such as payors and regulators who are concerned about quality of care to have a better understanding of the patient's situation and future plans and expectations. Thus, as nursing facility care becomes more complex, the role of physicians in the nursing facility becomes even more essential.

References

[1] Lawhorne LW, Walker G, Zweig SC, et al. Who cares for Missouri's Medicaid nursing home residents? Characteristics of attending physicians [see comment]. J Am Geriatr Soc 1993; 41(4):454–8.
[2] Besdine RW, Rubenstein LZ, Cassel C. Nursing home residents need physicians' services [editorial]. Ann Intern Med 1994;120:616–8.
[3] Kemper P, Murtaugh CM. Lifetime use of nursing home care. N Engl J Med 1991;324: 595–600.

[4] Lascaratos J, Kalantzis G, Poulakou-Rebelakou E. Nursing homes for the old ('Gerocomeia') in Byzantium (324–1453 AD). Gerontology 2004;50(2):113–7.

[5] Robben PB. Older chronic patients and their care provisions in the first half of the twentieth century. Tijdschr Gerontol Geriatr 1998;29(4):168–76 [in Dutch].

[6] Fleming KC, Evans JM, Chutka DS. A cultural and economic history of old age in America [see comment]. Mayo Clin Proc 2003;78(7):914–21.

[7] MMWR Morb Mortal Wkly Rep Feb 14, 2003;(52)6:101–4, 106.

[8] United States Census Bureau. Population division. 2004.

[9] Vital Health Statistics. The national nursing home survey: 1997 summary. Series 13 (No. 147).

[10] Cutler DM. Disability and the future of Medicare. N Engl J Med 2003;349:1084–5.

[11] Congdon JG, Magilvy JK. Rural nursing homes: a housing option for older adults. Geriatr Nurs 1998;19(3):157–9.

[12] Muramatsu N, Lee SY, Alexander JA. Hospital provision of institutional long-term care: pattern and correlates. Gerontologist 2000;40(5):557–67.

[13] Evashwick C, Swan JH, Smith P. Geriatric services offered by hospitals: predicting services by internal and external community characteristics. Home Health Care Serv Q 2001;19(3): 19–33.

[14] Dimant J. Roles and responsibilities of attending physicians in skilled nursing facilities [see comment]. J Am Med Dir Assoc 2003;4(4):231–43.

[15] United States Senate Special Committee on Aging. Developments in aging: 1997 and 1998. Washington, DC: 2000.

[16] Long-term care rules and regulations. Available at: http://www2.state.ga.us. Accessed February 27, 2005.

[17] Centers for Medicare and Medicaid Services. Available at: http://www.cms.hhs.gov/. Accessed February 27, 2005.

[18] Joint Commission on Accreditation of Healthcare Organizations. Available at: www.jcaho.org/index.htm. Accessed February 27, 2005.

[19] US Department of Labor Occupational Safety & Health Administration. Available at: www.osha.gov. Accessed February 27, 2005.

[20] Health Insurance Portability and Accountability Act of 1996. Available at: http://www.cms.hhs.gov/hipaa/. Accessed February 27, 2005.

[21] Pronvost PJ, Angus DC, Dorman T. Physician staffing patterns and clinical outcomes in critically ill patients: a systematic review. JAMA 2002;288:2151–62.

[22] Friedemann ML, Montgomery RJ, Maiberger B, et al. Family involvement in the nursing home: family-oriented practices and staff-family relationships. Res Nurs Health 1997;20(6): 527–37.

[23] Boise L, White D. The family's role in person-centered care: practice considerations. J Psychosoc Nurs Ment Health Serv 2004;42(5):12–20.

[24] Elon R. The nursing home medical director role in transition. J Am Geriatr Soc 1993;41: 131–5.

ELSEVIER
SAUNDERS

Prim Care Clin Office Pract
32 (2005) 811–828

PRIMARY CARE:
CLINICS IN
OFFICE PRACTICE

End-of-Life Care for Older Adults

Karen S. Ogle, MD*, Katrina Hopper, MS

*Department of Family Practice, College of Human Medicine, Michigan State University,
B110 Clinical Center, East Lansing, MI 48824, USA*

Changes in medicine and medical technology in the past half century have dramatically altered the way people die. A hundred years ago, infectious diseases were the major cause of death and the average age of death was 48 years [1]. But by the end of the twentieth century, chronic disease had become by far the predominant cause of death in America [1]. People today live to a much more advanced age, often with ongoing illness.

One role of the physician is to make such long life possible and to help assure that the life being prolonged can remain active, productive, and meaningful. However, despite all the technology at our disposal, death is still the inevitable consequence of most chronic diseases. There usually comes a time in the course of such illnesses when neither cure nor pro-longation of life can be a primary, or even reasonable, goal of care. This fact does not mean, however, that the physician has no further role. Physicians, typically primary care physicians, have a vital and valuable part to play in the care of patients who are nearing the end of their lives. Maximizing quality of life and providing effective symptom relief then become the most important goals of care.

The elderly comprise most of those in need of palliative and end-of-life care [2]. Nearly 2.5 million people died in the United States in 2002, and three quarters of those deaths occurred in those aged 65 years and over [3]. Five of the six leading causes of death in this age group were chronic illnesses, the conditions most likely to benefit from palliative care [4]. The elderly also represent the most rapidly growing segment of the population, with those aged 65 years and over expected to more than double from 2000 to 2030, when they will constitute 20% of the population. And the number of people aged 85 years and older is expected to more than double by 2030, and more than double again by 2050 [5]. Thus the need for palliative care for older adults will continue to rise at a rapid rate.

---

* Corresponding author.
  E-mail address: ogle@msu.edu (K.S. Ogle).

0095-4543/05/$ - see front matter © 2005 Elsevier Inc. All rights reserved.
doi:10.1016/j.pop.2005.06.005

Life-limiting chronic illnesses include advanced cancer, neurodegenerative diseases, and organ or system failure. Cancer increases in frequency and rate of death with advancing years. The incidence of neurodegenerative diseases and advanced pulmonary, cardiovascular, and renal diseases also increases dramatically with age. These noncancer diagnoses often have less predictable trajectories [6], making accurate prognostication and definite identification of the time called "end of life" more difficult [6–8]. "Diagnosing dying" is a complex challenge, requiring clinical insights beyond those related to traditional diagnosis and treatment, and advanced communication skills to allow the physician to share those insights with patients and families [8,9].

An additional challenge is the decrease in cognitive function experienced by some older patients, whether this means full-blown dementia or reduced capacity for decision making for other reasons. Patient incapacity and the need for family members to take on all or part of the decision-making responsibility put even greater demands on the physician [10,11]. The article by Brody elsewhere in this issue provides a more detailed discussion of decision-making capacity.

But challenges can lead to great rewards in the lives of terminally ill patients and their families. By making end-of-life care a vital component of office-based geriatrics, the physician can supply early assistance with future care planning, help patients and families identify goals of care, provide intensive/active symptom management, and address important life closure issues [12]. Few physicians have had extensive training in how to manage these complex situations, and they may react to them with avoidance or indecision. But the skills for addressing the common concerns of geriatric patients at the end of life are easily developed [6,13]. This article addresses:

- Goals of care
- Communication with patients and families
- Coordination of services
- Symptom management, including physical, psychosocial, and spiritual symptoms
- The active dying process
- Grief and bereavement

Goals of care

The many possible goals of medical care range from prevention of disease and prolongation of life to symptom control and helping patients to achieve a "good death." It is important to realize that different, and even conflicting, goals of care for a patient can coexist. Such goals also do not remain static; their identification and reassessment is an ongoing process over the course of a patient's illness, especially as patients near the end of life because priorities and goals often change as symptoms grow more severe or when the patient comes to understand that proposed treatments have minimal chance of prolonging life [14].

Health care providers should revisit goals of care regularly, particularly during points of crisis or transition. Four major areas of change in a patient's life should trigger a reassessment of the goals of care [15,16]:

A change in the patient's health status (eg, worsened prognosis or unexpected recovery)

A change in the patient's treatment setting (eg, hospital to nursing home, or vice versa)

A change in treatment options that results from disease progression or unresponsiveness to current therapy

The expressed preference of a patient to change the goals of care

The family or proxy decision maker usually should be present when discussing goals of care with the terminally ill patient. If the patient later becomes unable to make decisions regarding medical care, those entrusted with decision-making responsibility will have additional insight and knowledge of the patient's goals for end-of-life care. Physicians also need to be aware that focusing decision making on the patient alone is not always the norm. In various cultures or subcultures, decision making involves the whole family, with a specific assignment of roles within the family (such as in many Asian or Hispanic cultures). Physicians should be sensitive to patients' and families' cultural contexts [11,17].

Advance directives are valuable in identifying proxy decision makers and do-not-resuscitate (DNR) status, and, ideally, advance care planning will cover a range of situations and care options that the patient or proxy decision maker might face as a chronic disease progresses. But there is no way to anticipate every possibility and permutation in the course of illness, so advance directives will provide only limited information about a patient's goals and wishes at the end of life. The conversations that elicit a patient's choices for advance directives are often more important than the legal document itself [18]. As with setting the goals of care, it is wise for the proxy to be present during these conversations so that he or she may be better equipped to speak on the patient's behalf in situations that have been anticipated and those that have not. Advance care planning should be reviewed whenever a patient experiences a crisis or point of transition, as outlined earlier. It is common for a patient's preferences to change during the course of a life-threatening chronic illness.

Communication with patients and families

Families play an important role in the well-being of those who are dying, but often suffer emotionally, spiritually, and financially as they care for the patient [19]. They may feel hopelessness, anger, guilt, and powerlessness when they cannot relieve the suffering of their terminally ill family member.

Family conflicts may resurface in the face of a terminal illness, and any emotional tension that exists between the caregivers and patient could impede care. It is helpful for physicians to observe how patients and their families communicate and to be sensitive to conflict and cultural influences. Physicians can provide support for patients and their families by allowing them to express their emotions and concerns and by referring them to appropriate counselors or support groups when needed [14,16].

Negotiating goals of care with terminally ill patients and their families can be a challenging task. A stepwise protocol [11,17,20] helps guide physicians through the process:

Create the right setting
Determine what the patient and family know
Ask how much they know and want to discuss with you
Explore what they are expecting or hoping for
Suggest realistic goals
Respond empathically
Make a plan and follow through

Coordination of care

Good end-of-life care cannot be provided by a physician alone. When possible, an interdisciplinary team should conduct an assessment and craft a plan that meets the full range of spiritual, emotional, and physical needs of a patient at the end of life [7,11]. Primary care physicians are often skilled at coordinating care between specialists and other health care providers, but coordinating an interdisciplinary team in the care of a dying patient can be a more daunting task. Fortunately, there are resources to assist physicians.

Hospice services are the most commonly used resource for terminally ill patients. Hospice refers to a philosophy of care and not any specific infrastructure. Hospice care is provided by an interdisciplinary team, and focuses primarily on symptom control and psychologic and spiritual support for dying patients and their families. In the United State, these services are generally provided by public or private agencies in home-care programs, long-term care facilities, or special residential facilities. Hospice care is defined by the Medicare hospice benefit, which requires a physician's certification that a patient is expected to live 6 months or less. Because it can be difficult to predict the life expectancy of elderly patients who have chronic diseases, many of them are never referred to hospice care, whereas others receive hospice services for only a short time before their deaths. For older adults who have a noncancer diagnosis with a less predictable trajectory to death, it may be best if the physician asked, "Would I be surprised if this patient died in the next 6 months?" Many have found this question to be useful in identifying patients who should be considered for end-of-life care. There is widespread agreement that earlier identification of patients who would benefit from hospice care, and earlier admission to hospice programs, would greatly enhance the quality of end-of-life care in the United States [7,21].

Most people express a preference for dying at home, and family members can often support that wish [18]. But various factors may make it impossible to deliver quality end-of-life care in the patient's home. Hospice care can also be provided in nursing facilities, and a growing number of nursing homes have instituted palliative care protocols for the care of residents at the end of life [8,22]. Patients who have less intensive-care needs may be suited for placement in an assisted living facility, where hospice services can also be provided. In addition, many hospices have residential units designed to care for patients who require intensive symptom management or have physical care needs that cannot be met in other settings. For patients for whom hospice is not a suitable choice, other community resources can be mobilized, including home health agencies or area agencies on aging [23]. The use of community resources is covered in more detail in the article by Holmes elsewhere in this issue.

Symptom management

Symptom management refers not only to physical symptoms that need to be addressed, but also to psychosocial concerns and spiritual distress. It is important to recognize that these three areas are interdependent, and that effective care of the whole person requires attention to all three in an integrated fashion. Primary care physicians can reduce or alleviate the burden of suffering in all of these areas. In most cases, the physician will want to coordinate care with other professionals who are integral to the patient's care, usually nurses, social workers, and home health aides. Many older patients will also appreciate the opportunity to meet with spiritual care professionals. Some patients may benefit from consultation with experts in palliative medicine or geriatrics or professionals who have more advanced psychosocial expertise, such as neuropsychologists or geriatric psychiatrists.

Specific details about symptom management are beyond the scope of this article, but the Further Readings section identifies resources for further information in all three areas.

Physical symptoms

The most common physical symptoms in terminally ill elderly patients include pain, dyspnea, nausea and vomiting, constipation, and fatigue. Certain symptoms are common no matter what the cause of death: nearly three quarters of all dying patients experience pain, and half have difficulty breathing and loss of appetite [24]. In most cases, the primary care physician can substantially relieve the burden of suffering from these symptoms. Consultation may be required in a few cases.

Evidence suggests that physical symptom management may be even more important in elderly dying patients than in others [10,18]. Many symptoms near the time of death, no matter what the cause of death, are more common with advancing age. Those aged 85 years and older are more than twice as likely as those younger than age 55 to experience confusion (52% versus 21%) or loss of bladder control (51% versus 24%) [24]. Elderly patients are also more likely to experience dizziness or loss of bowel control.

Pain

Pain is a common symptom in older adults in general, with estimates as high as 50% of older adults experiencing major pain [25]. But although pain is widespread in elderly people, pain relief often is not achieved. It has been shown repeatedly that elderly people are at greater risk for inadequate analgesia than younger persons. Women and non-Caucasians are also at increased risk for poor pain relief. When older patients suffer from advanced illness, particular attention is required to ensure pain relief. Rates of pain in metastatic cancer range from 60% to 90%, and pain is also common in the advanced stages of many other chronic diseases, with rates from 50% to 80% reported. Pain may be caused by the disease process itself, co-morbidities, or the medical treatments provided.

Pain assessment should include a thorough history, relevant physical examination, and assessment of functional status. Atypical presentations of pain are common in elder patients, and may include confusion, fatigue, withdrawal, and depression. Inquiring specifically about pain is even more important in elderly patients than in the general population. The multiple comorbidities of elderly patients often complicate the assessment of pain, and pain from multiple sources is common.

A standardized approach should be used to assess pain and to evaluate the severity of the pain. Such an approach can also enhance communication about the effectiveness of interventions used to relieve pain. Standard tools include the numeric rating scale, the visual analog scale, and the faces scale. Special tools have been developed for pain assessment in cognitively impaired patients [18]. Cognitively impaired older patients who are unable to report their pain pose a particular challenge in pain assessment. Self-report may need to be replaced by careful observation of behaviors and facial expressions. Pain should always be considered in the differential diagnosis of agitation or withdrawal in older adults who are cognitively impaired.

Pharmacologic treatment is required for pain in most terminally ill older adults. Acetaminophen is well tolerated and generally recognized as the drug of choice for mild pain in elderly patients. The adverse effects of non-steroidal anti-inflammatory drugs, including cyclooxygenase-2 inhibitors are greatly increased in elderly people, and most experts prefer to avoid their use where possible [26,27]. Adjuvant analgesics, including antidepressants and anticonvulsants, can be considered, but a high degree of caution regarding adverse effects and potential for interactions with other drugs must be exercised in the elderly population. Corticosteroids should also be considered for relief of refractory pain in the terminally ill, where the risk for serious adverse effects may be outweighed by the potential benefit. Corticosteroids are particularly likely to be beneficial in pain caused by bone metastases and neuropathic causes [26,28].

Opioids are the mainstay of therapy for relief of moderate to severe pain. They should be titrated upward until pain relief is achieved or unmanageable adverse effects are manifested. Titration should be done with special care in elderly patients because of their altered pharmacokinetics and increased sensitivity to adverse effects. In addition, one should consider the possibility that longer-than-usual dosing intervals may be needed. Most patients will do best on regularly scheduled or around-the-clock dosing, with rescue or as needed (PRN) medication available for episodes of breakthrough pain.

Oral administration is the simplest and preferred route for most elderly patients. Initial treatment and titration to pain relief should use immediate release preparations of opioids. However, once good pain relief has been achieved, sustained release preparations will provide equivalent analgesia with dosing at substantially reduced intervals (every 8–12 hours). Rescue medication should be maintained in the immediate release form.

Some patients will not be able to use the oral route for various reasons (eg, difficulty swallowing, gastrointestinal obstruction). Fentanyl is the only opioid currently available commercially for transdermal delivery. Transdermal patches are effective for many people, but elderly patients may have more erratic responses because of alterations in skin integrity, subcutaneous fat, and serum albumin [26]. Alternatively, compounding pharmacists may prepare cream or gel versions of opioids for transdermal administration. Morphine gel has also been used as an effective topical analgesic treatment for painful skin lesions, including pressure ulcers [29]. Opioids may also be administered rectally, either using ready-made suppositories or by rectal administration of immediate or sustained release oral preparations.

Parenteral administration of opioids may be needed in some patients. Subcutaneous administration (either continuous or intermittent) may be highly effective, and intravenous infusions are used in many patients who have pre-existing ports from earlier therapies. Intramuscular (IM) injections should be discouraged. In addition to causing pain, absorption from IM injections is erratic, and the analgesia achieved is generally no better than with less invasive routes [26,28]. A small percentage of patients will require epidural or intrathecal delivery of analgesics, usually because of refractory systemic adverse effects from other routes [28].

The specific opioid may be chosen by availability of the preferred route or that of sustained release preparations. Oxycodone and hydromorphone have shorter half-lives and lower potential for accumulation of toxic metabolites than morphine, so they may be preferred in elderly patients. In general, meperidine should not be used because of its poor oral absorption and neurotoxic active metabolite, particularly problematic in older patients who have reduced renal function [26].

Nonpharmacologic methods may be useful adjunctive measures for pain relief in elderly patients. Massage, exercise, positioning, and application of heat or cold can contribute to relief in some cases. Mind–body techniques, such as relaxation or imagery, may also be helpful, but the physician should take care not to send the mistaken message that their usefulness means the pain is "all in the patient's head." Elderly patients vary in their receptivity to these techniques [26].

Dyspnea

Dyspnea, or breathlessness, is a highly distressing symptom common in many end-stage disease processes. Although reversible causes should be sought and aggressively managed, dyspnea unfortunately remains a significant symptom for many individuals even after maximal disease treatment. Opioids, particularly morphine, provide highly effective relief of dyspnea for most patients. Benzodiazepines, and to a lesser extent, phenothiazines, have been used to treat dyspnea. There is no clear evidence as to which category of medication will be most effective in any given patient, and clinical judgment combined with therapeutic trials is the best approach. The use of oxygen is common in treatment of dyspnea, but it is not always effective. Hypoxemia does not necessarily correlate with the subjective symptom of dyspnea, and its correction may not produce symptom relief. The drawbacks of oxygen therapy include cost, the intrusive and noisy apparatus, restrictions on activity, and difficulties in keeping tubing or masks in place in many elderly patients. The relative benefits and drawbacks should be weighed for each individual, and a therapeutic trial to assess benefit considered. Use of oxygen only on a PRN basis should also be considered. Nonpharmacologic interventions for dyspnea, such as positioning, dehumidification of ambient air, the use of fans, and soothing environmental changes, are often highly effective adjuncts to pharmacologic treatment. Calm reassurance by the physician or other health care professional is also of great therapeutic benefit when combined with other interventions.

Nausea and vomiting

Nausea and vomiting may be caused by the underlying medical conditions or by their treatments (eg, opioids). Different causes of nausea can be addressed in particular ways. For example, gastric stasis may be treated with prokinetic medications, such as metoclopramide. Antihistamines, like meclizine, may relieve movement-related nausea. Much of the nausea that occurs at the end of life is mediated by stimulation of the chemoreceptor trigger zone, and treatment may include dopamine antagonists, such as phenothiazines or butyrophenones, or 5HT antagonists, such as ondansetron. Unfortunately, many elderly patients are particularly vulnerable to the adverse sedative, anticholinergic, and extrapyramidal effects of these medications, which limits their usefulness. A common exacerbating factor is caregiver insistence that patients who do not have an appetite should nevertheless eat. Physician counseling about this problem is reviewed below.

Dehydration and weight loss

Although these conditions are not typically symptomatic, they are often of great concern to family members, who may worry that their loved one will "die of thirst" or "starve to death." Concerned family are undoubtedly also influenced by the fact that feeding is seen as a sign of love, and they might worry that withholding food and hydration will hasten death. However, nonoral administration of fluids or calories in a dying patient does not prolong life. On the contrary, it may make the life that remains less comfortable by increasing congestion and swelling, or by possibly enhancing tumor growth in cancer patients. Patients and family should be reassured that it is natural to lose interest in eating in advanced illness, and that taking in less fluid and fewer calories can actually help make the patient more comfortable. It does not cause suffering and can ease the physical part of the dying process. Reassurance from the physician is usually well received and can be an important source of relief and comfort [30,31].

Patients who are dehydrated in the advanced stages of illness may experience dry mouth, but this is not related to thirst, and any discomfort can be relieved with the use of ice chips or a wet cloth.

Fatigue

Fatigue is another common symptom, but regrettably not one that is easily relieved. Although correctible factors, including depression, should be sought and addressed where appropriate, persistent fatigue is common in advanced illness. Letting patients know that fatigue is not unusual can be valuable for them and their families, who may interpret this symptom as a sign the patient is "giving up." Counseling regarding energy conservation strategies, including identification and pacing of high-priority activities, may be helpful. Medical interventions have limited effectiveness, but carefully selected patients may benefit from a trial of therapy with psychostimulants. There is modest research evidence of benefit with methylphenidate, and anecdotal reports of positive effects from modafinil.

Constipation

Constipation is common in elderly people, and is further increased by advanced illness and debilitation. It is also a frequent adverse effect of many drugs, including opioids and those with anti-cholinergic side effects. Even in the absence of such drugs, decreased gastrointestinal motility can occur near the end of life, and the clinician should always be aware of the possibility that ileus, mechanical obstruction, or metabolic abnormalities can lead to a decrease in the number of bowel movements.

A common error in the treatment of constipation is failure to titrate to an effective dose of a single agent. Regular administration of stimulant laxatives (eg, senna, bisacodyl) or osmotic agents (eg, milk of magnesia, sorbitol, lactulose, polyethylene glycol) is often necessary for management of constipation in the terminally ill. Opioids are a major cause of constipation, and as Cicely Saunders [32], the founder of the modern hospice movement, has stated, "The hand that writes the opioid prescription should also write the laxative." Preliminary studies have shown encouraging results relieving constipation with oral administration of opioid antagonists (in particular, methylnaltrexone, which does not cross the blood–brain barrier).

Skin care

Problems with the skin are most effectively addressed through prevention. The patient should be bathed routinely, with thorough drying to reduce the risk for maceration. Topical antibiotics or antifungals can be used as needed. Pressure increases the risk for ischemia and subsequent skin breakdown. Standard nursing techniques will greatly reduce this risk, although it is important to recognize that the skin is just one more organ system prone to failure in the very late stages of life. When elevation is not required for social interaction or symptom relief, keeping the head of the bed lowered can minimize sacral pressure. Bony prominences should be protected with hydrocolloid dressings. Despite short-term discomfort with turning, most patients are more comfortable overall with regular turning, which also helps to minimize skin breakdown. A "logroll" technique should be used, and a draw sheet will reduce shearing forces. The care of skin wounds that do develop should focus more on comfort than healing. Minimizing dressing changes, use of nonadherent dressings, and attention to odor management are ways to promote comfort [33].

Psychosocial concerns

Psychosocial sources of distress include anxiety, depression, and family needs. All are common issues during the course of an advanced illness, and need not be "medicalized" for all patients. Nonetheless, a substantial number of patients will have sufficient distress to merit interventions beyond simple support.

Anxiety

Anxiety is a common response to the uncertainties involved in confronting one's impending death, but it may also be fueled by poorly relieved physical symptoms, such as pain or dyspnea. In addition, it may be a primary psychiatric problem, even one of longstanding duration. Non-pharmacologic interventions include counseling, social services, and directly addressing any specific fears about what happens in the dying process. When pharmacologic management is also needed, chronic anxiety often responds well to a selective serotonin reuptake inhibitor. Benzodiazepines may be needed for some patients, but their potential to increase the risk for falls and delirium should be carefully considered.

Depression

Most patients facing a terminal diagnosis experience a range of sad, angry, helpless, and even hopeless feelings. For many, however, these feelings are temporary, intermittent, or moderate in intensity. Clinical depression is not always easy to identify in terminally ill patients, as many of the standard markers (eg, poor appetite, sleep disturbance, fatigue) may be caused by the underlying illness [34]. Research has suggested that simply asking the question "Are you depressed?" can be an effective method of screening [35]. Dysphoria and anhedonia are also more specific signs of depression. As with anxiety, treatment of depression may include non-pharmacologic and pharmacologic interventions. Psychologic counseling, along with spiritual support, may be valuable, and antidepressants, combined with renewed attention to meticulous management of other physical symptoms, may also contribute to relief for many patients. In severe cases, and with patients very close to death, there may be benefit in a trial of psychostimulants, which will provide faster response to therapy. Standard antidepressants can be started concurrently where appropriate. Mirtazapine may be a particularly useful antidepressant in advanced illness, because of its common side effects of enhanced appetite and improved sleep [26]. A more detailed description of the recognition, assessment, and management of depression can be found in the article by Lawhorne elsewhere in this issue.

Spiritual issues

Regardless of previous spiritual beliefs or practices, most people have spiritual or existential concerns when facing the imminent end of life. Many elderly people address these concerns in the context of an established religion, but increasing numbers will do so in other contexts. Religion and belief in God are not necessarily part of spirituality, which can be defined broadly as an involvement in that which is beyond our normal senses, and which gives life meaning [9,36].

Research suggests that patients want physicians to inquire more about this aspect of their lives, but the extent to which individual physicians are comfortable discussing matters of spirituality varies. At a minimum, physicians should ask about possible spiritual concerns and should be able to validate common questions that arise, such as "Why is this happening to me?" "What has my life meant—to me and to others?" and "What happens to us after we die?" The physician need not provide answers to these questions, but can help immensely by acknowledging their importance and the frequency with which they are asked at this stage of life. Physicians should not feel that they are expected to pursue discussions beyond their level of comfort; neither should they take such questions as a license to impose their own beliefs or to proselytize. Spiritual care providers may be available from the patient's own tradition or from hospice programs, hospitals, and nursing facilities. Most chaplains are skilled at working with patients from diverse backgrounds and on each patient's own terms [34,36].

The active dying process

Care during the last hours of life should be a core competency of every physician, and anticipatory guidance should be provided to all patients and their family members. Guidance about what to expect helps reduce fear and anxiety about the process while also increasing the patient's confidence. Hospice programs can be invaluable sources of support in providing this guidance, and physicians may also find it useful to devote a family meeting to the topic. Managing the active dying process requires careful planning with the patient, the family, and the care team, with attention to communication plans and the expected symptom management needs. This preparation should also include plans for care of the body after death. Common patient and family guidance needs are outlined in Box 1.

Death generally comes as a consequence of widespread systemic change rather than the failure of a single system or organ [9]. Homeostasis in the body is lost and catabolic processes develop, leading to progressive and irreversible decline. Understanding this fact helps in addressing the active dying process more effectively [21]. The individual's ability to distribute, metabolize, and use drugs may be rapidly impaired, and rapid changes also occur in physiologic parameters. Anticipatory treatment provides the most effective symptom management during the active dying process [33]. All nonessential medications and treatments should be stopped, and for those that are continued, the route of delivery should be re-evaluated. When patients are not able to take oral medications, many medications can still be given by buccal, rectal, or subcutaneous routes; the best route will vary with the individual patient and family. The family should be reassured about hydration issues.

Pain management remains an important goal, but pain may actually decrease at this stage because of decreasing neurologic activity and the buildup of endogenous chemicals with analgesic properties. The major metabolites of opioids are cleared by the kidney, and thus are likely to

---

Box 1. Patient and family guidance needs to prepare for the dying process

Patient and family tasks
- Identify sources of available health care support; consider use of hospice care.
- Anticipate symptom management needs and prepare family.
- Facilitate life closure needs.
- Plan for rituals and rites: funeral or memorial service.
- Plan for desired place of death; facilitate home death or plan for other sites.

Family education
- What are common behaviors near death (eg, communication in metaphor and visits from deceased friends and relatives).
- What are the signs that death is near.
- How to recognize that death has occurred.
- What to do after death occurs.

---

accumulate during this phase. The potential for adverse neuroexcitatory effects, which increase the frequency and severity of terminal agitation and delirium, has led to the recommendation that routine administration be discontinued, and any signs of pain be managed with breakthrough (PRN) doses only [33].

Loss of the ability to swallow and manage secretions is common in the active dying phase. Secretions may accumulate in the oropharynx and the tracheobronchial tree, leading to gurgling or rattling sounds that may be distressing to the family (the so-called death rattle). Anticipatory management is the most effective approach, combined with reassurance to the family that these sounds do not reflect actual patient distress. Started early, anticholinergic medication will minimize the accumulation of such secretions, but will not dry up already established secretions. Postural drainage may be helpful, but suctioning should be discouraged because of its stimulating and painful effects [26,33].

Terminal delirium may present with confusion or restlessness, and may develop into a highly agitated state that is distressing to patient and family. Remediable causes of agitation that may be suspected, such as unrelieved pain or a distended bladder, should be quickly assessed and addressed. Treatment should then focus on muscle relaxation and sedation, which will minimize distress for the patient, family members, and others in attendance. Benzodiazepines are highly effective in relieving this syndrome, with their sedating, muscle-relaxing, and anticonvulsant properties. They can be given and rapidly titrated through the buccal or subcutaneous route.

Occasionally, these agents have a paradoxical effect, and neuroleptics may be required instead. Nonpharmacologic treatment is also valuable: dimmed lighting, soothing music, and gentle touch can be helpful. Family members may also benefit from these strategies. Those attending the deathbed can be encouraged to speak soothingly to the patient. Family members can help ease the final passage by giving the dying person permission to let go, and by giving assurance that those left behind will be all right [26,33].

Other common changes near death, such as mottled skin color and irregular breathing patterns, should be discussed with families. Most hospice programs have handouts that describe these signs of impending death, along with signs that death has occurred.

Immediately after death

When death occurs, the primary focus of care becomes the family. Friends and family members should be encouraged to spend as much time as they wish with the body, allowing them to begin to absorb this profound change in their lives and to say goodbye. Where appropriate, brief preparation of the body may make this process easier for family: removing all catheters, tubes, and machinery; cleaning up any body fluids released; and placing the body in a natural and relaxed position.

Regulations regarding pronouncement of death vary according to state, and physicians should be aware of relevant local and state regulations. Generally, a physician is not required to pronounce death in a case where it was expected, and the hospice nurse may do so. Similarly, restrictions by funeral directors may vary regarding when the death certificate must be signed by the physician. In most communities, there are no specific regulations about when the body must be removed. Families should be encouraged to take as much time as they desire with the body; considerable evidence suggests that spending a longer time than is customary in American society may benefit the grief process.

Grief and bereavement

After the death, family members require time to absorb the loss and its impact on their lives. The acute phase of grief is often intense and requires considerable support. A phone call from the physician in the first few days after the loss is often deeply appreciated, and a condolence card is another welcome expression of support and recognition of the loss. Physicians who had a close relationship with the patient or family may also wish to attend visitation or funeral services. Although most families do not expect this, they are frequently moved by it, and the physician may also find it beneficial for personal closure.

Experts describe four related tasks of grieving that follow the death of an important person in one's life [33]:

Step 1. Recognize the loss.
Step 2. Experience the pain of the loss.
Step 3. Recognize the significance and meaning of the loss.
Step 4. Reinvest in life; discover what is left.

These steps do not necessarily proceed in a linear fashion from one to the next. The first task has been described as the recognition of the loss. Deeply involved family caregivers often find this step surprisingly difficult, and physicians may hear comments like "I can't believe he is really gone" or "I just can't seem to take it in." The second task in moving through the process of grief is experiencing the pain of the loss. This may be very difficult, and physicians may want to alleviate this suffering with medications. But although pharmacotherapy may be needed for highly agitated, destructive, or severely depressed reactions, drugs should be prescribed with caution. There is significant risk that extended use of medication will prolong the grief process and complicate its eventual resolution.

A further task for those who grieve is to absorb and recognize the significance of the loss and its multidimensional effects on their lives. Finally, bereaved individuals must find ways to reinvest in living and determine what aspects of life—as it was before the death and as it is now—can give it meaning. This phase often has a deep spiritual dimension [33,36].

Modern American society tends to set expectations about the grief process that are at odds with human nature and need. The "acceptable" timeframe for grief is far too short, and the expectations for "getting over it" are unrealistic. Studies of grieving adults show that grief is often an active process for 1 to 2 years after the loss, and that many individuals describe a process of learning to live with the loss as opposed to a "recovery" from it. Normalizing and validating these common responses can be helpful to the bereaved, especially when it comes with the powerful imprimatur of the physician. At the same time, the physician should remain alert for signs of complicated grief that requires more expert management than most physicians are trained to provide. These signs may include intense reactions that do not subside or fluctuate over time; suppressed or postponed reactions; exaggerated or destructive behaviors; and lack of awareness of feelings or behaviors. People experiencing complicated grief need the assistance of a professional who has special expertise in this area. Physicians should identify such professionals in the community and offer referrals to patients who have complicated grief.

Grief support services may be available through local hospices, even for those who did not use the hospice services in many cases. Community-based groups also offer grief support, and the surviving spouse of an elderly patient may particularly benefit from participation.

Summary

   Caring for elderly patients and their families at the end of life gives physicians the opportunity to have a meaningful impact on the lives of others. By expanding our clinical expertise beyond the arena of cure and the preservation of life, we can discover new ways to encounter our patients as full human beings and to share a profound life passage that many of us might otherwise ignore. The skills that are needed to enter this new arena are well within the grasp of the office-based clinician, and physicians who employ them are rewarded with the fulfillment of knowing they have provided an invaluable service at a time of greatest need.

Further readings

Bandolier. Available at: http://www.jr2.ox.ac.uk/bandolier/index.html.
Completing a life—a resource for taking charge, finding comfort & reaching closure. Available at: http://www.completingalife.msu.edu.
Doyle D, Hanks G, Cherny NI, et al. Oxford textbook of palliative medicine. 3rd edition. New York: Oxford University Press; 2003.
Educating physicians in end-of-life care. Available at: http://epec.net.
Growth House: a guide to death, dying, grief, bereavement and end-of-life care. Available at: http://www.growthhouse.org. Accessed June 30, 2005.
Morrison RS, Meier DE. Palliative care. N Engl J Med 2004;350(25):2582–90.
Morrison RS, Meier DE, Capello C. Geriatric palliative care. New York: Oxford University Press; 2003.
National Cancer Institute. PDQ cancer information summaries. Available at: http://www.cancer.gov/cancerinfo/pdq/supportivecare.
Neuberger J. Caring for dying people of different faiths. London: Radcliffe Medical Press; 2004.
Pain medicine and palliative care. Available at: http://stoppain.org.
Puchalski CM, Dorff RE, Hendi IY. Spirituality, religion, and healing in palliative care. Clin Geriatr Med 2004;20:689–714.
Shaarey Zadek cancer pain and palliative care reference database. Available at: http://chernydatabase.org.
Article series in JAMA: "Perspectives on Care at the Close of Life."

References

[1] Administration on Aging, US Department of Health and Human Services. A profile of older Americans: 2002. Available at: http://www.aoa.gov/prof/statistics/profile/profiles 2002.asp. Accessed January 31, 2005.
[2] Brock D, Foley D. Demography and epidemiology of dying in the US with emphasis on deaths of older persons. Hosp J 1998;13:49–60.
[3] National Center for Health Statistics. Number of deaths, death rates, and age-adjusted death rates by race and sex; United States, 1950, 1960, 1970, 1980–2002. Available at: http://www.cdc.gov/nchs/fastasts/pdf/mortality/nvrs53_05t0.1.pdf. Accessed June 30, 2005.
[4] Federal Interagency Forum on Aging. Related statistics older Americans 2004: key indicators of well-being, indicator 14, mortality. Available at: http://www.agingstats.gov/chartbook2004/health_status.pdf. Accessed January 31, 2005.

[5] Federal Interagency Forum on Aging. Related statistics older Americans 2004: key indicators of well-being, indicator 13, life expectancy. Available at: http://www.agingstats. gov/chartbook2004/tables-population.html. Accessed January 31, 2005.

[6] Murray SA, Boyd K, Sheikh A, et al. Developing primary palliative care: people with terminal conditions should be able to die at home with dignity. BMJ 2004;329:1056–7.

[7] Lynne J. Serving patients who may die soon and their families: the role of hospice and other service. JAMA 2001;285:925–32.

[8] Weitzen S, Teno JM, Fennell M, et al. Factors associated with site of death: a national study of where people die. Med Care 2003;2:323–35.

[9] Ellershaw J, Ward C. Care of the dying patient: the last hours or days of life. BMJ 2003;326: 30–4.

[10] Evers M, Meier DE, Morrison S. Assessing differences in care needs and service utilization in geriatric palliative care patients. J Pain Symptom Manage 2002;23(5):424–32.

[11] Morrison RS, Meier DE. Palliative care. N Engl J Med 2004;350(25):2582–90.

[12] Seymour J, Clark D. Palliative care and geriatric medicine: shared concerns, shared challenges. Palliat Med 2001;15:269–70.

[13] Farber NJ, Urban SY, Collier VU, et al. Frequency and perceived competence in providing palliative care to terminally ill patients: a survey of primary care physicians. J Pain Symptom Manage 2004;28(4):364–72.

[14] Larson DG, Tobin DR. End of life conversations: evolving practice and theory. JAMA 2000; 284(12):1573–8.

[15] Block SD, Billings JA. Patient request to hasten death: evaluation and management in terminal care. Arch Intern Med 1994;154:2039–47.

[16] Della Santina C, Bernstein RH. Whole patient assessment, goal planning, and inflection points: their role in achieving quality end-of-life care. Clin Geriatr Med 2004;20:595–620.

[17] Education for physicians on end-of-life care: Module 7 Goals of Care. Chicago: AMA; 1999. p. 1–16.

[18] Sheehan DK, Schirm V. End of life care of older adults: debunking some common misconceptions about dying in old age. Am J Nurs 2003;103(11):48–58.

[19] Rabow M, Hauser J, Adams J. Supporting family caregivers at the end of life: "they don't know what they don't know". JAMA 2004;291:483–91.

[20] Buckman R. How to break bad news: a guide for health care professionals. Baltimore (MD): Johns Hopkins University Press; 1992.

[21] Stevenson J, Abernathy AP, Miller C, et al. Managing comorbidities in patients at the end of life. BMJ 2004;329:909–12.

[22] Miller SC, Teno JM, Mor V. Hospice and palliative care in nursing homes. Clin Geriatr Med 2004;20:717–34.

[23] Ryan SD, Tuuk M, Lee M. Pace and hospice: two models of palliative care on the verge of collaboration. Clin Geriatr Med 2004;20:783–94.

[24] Seal C, Cartwright A. The year before death. Brookfield (VT): Ashgate Publishing Company; 1994.

[25] Ferrell BA. Pain management. Clin Geriatr Med 2000;16:853–74.

[26] Brown JA, Von Roenn JH. Symptom management in the older adult. Clin Geriatr Med 2004;20:621–40.

[27] The management of chronic pain in older persons. AGS panel on chronic pain in older persons. American Geriatrics Society. Geriatrics 1998;53(3):S8–24.

[28] Cleary JF, Carbone PD. Palliative medicine in the elderly. Cancer 1997;80(7):1335–47.

[29] Twillman RK, Long TD, Cathers TA, et al. Treatment of painful skin ulcers with topical opioids. J Pain Symptom Manage 1999;17(4):288–92.

[30] McCann RM, Hall WJ, Groth-Juncker A. Comfort care for terminally ill patients: the appropriate use of nutrition and hydration. JAMA 1994;272:1263–6.

[31] Billings JA. Comfort measures for the terminally ill: is dehydration painful? J Am Geriatr Soc 1985;33:808–10.

[32] Yuan CS, Foss JF, O'Connor M, et al. Effects of intravenous methylnaltrexone on opioid-induced gut motility and transit time changes in subjects receiving chronic methadone therapy: a pilot study. Pain 1999;83:631–5.

[33] Ferris FD. Last hours of living. Clin Geriatr Med 2004;20:641–67.

[34] Chochinov HM. Thinking outside the box: depression, hope and meaning at the end of life. J Palliat Med 2003;6:973–7.

[35] Chochinov Hm, Wilson KG, Enns M, et al. "Are you depressed?" screening for depression in the terminally ill. Am J Psychiatry 1997;154(5):674–6.

[36] Puchalski CM, Dorff RE, Hendi IY. Spirituality, religion, and healing in palliative care. Clin Geriatr Med 2004;20:689–714.

ELSEVIER
SAUNDERS

Prim Care Clin Office Pract
32 (2005) 829–853

PRIMARY CARE:
CLINICS IN
OFFICE PRACTICE

Appendices: Examples of Available Tools for Screening and Evaluation

1. Nutrition: determine your nutritional health checklist
2. Instrumental activities of daily living (IADL) scale
3. Cognition
   a. Clock drawing task
   b. Functional activities questionnaire
   c. Mini-mental state examination (MMSE)
   d. DSM-IV criteria for dementia
   e. DSM-IV criteria for delirium

4. Mobility
   a. Get up and go test
   b. Performance-oriented mobility screen

5. Psychologic function
   a. Geriatric depression scale
   b. DSM-IV criteria for major depression
   c. Cornell scale for depression in dementia

6. Alcohol
   a. Michigan alcoholism screening test—geriatric version (MAST-G)
   b. The CAGE questionnaire

7. Caregiver
   a. Zarit burden interview
   b. The caregiver strain questionnaire

8. Environment—home safety checklist

0095-4543/05/$ - see front matter © 2005 Elsevier Inc. All rights reserved.
doi:10.1016/j.pop.2005.06.012   *primarycare.theclinics.com*

Appendix 1: Nutrition

Determine your nutritional health checklist

	YES
I have an illness or condition that made me change the kind and/or amount of food that I eat.	2
I eat fewer than 2 meals per day.	3
I eat few fruits or vegetables or milk products.	2
I have 3 or more drinks of beer, liquor, or wine almost every day.	2
I have tooth or mouth problems that make it hard for me to eat.	2
I don't always have enough money to buy the food I need.	4
I eat alone most of the time.	1
I take 3 or more different prescribed or over-the-counter drugs a day.	1
Without wanting to, I have lost or gained 10 pounds in the last 6 months.	2
I am not always physically able to shop, cook, and/or feed myself.	2
Total	

Total your nutritional score. If it's:

0–2: **Good**. Recheck your nutritional score in 6 months.

3–5: **You are at moderate nutritional risk**. See what you can do to improve your eating habits and lifestyle. Your office on aging, senior nutritional program, senior citizen center, or health department can help. Recheck your nutritional score in 3 months.

6 or more: **You are at high nutritional risk**. Bring the checklist the next time you see your doctor, dietician, or other qualified health or social service professional. Talk with them about any problems you may have. Ask for help to improve your nutritional health.

Modified from American Academy of Family Physicians. Determine your nutritional health. Available at: http://www.aafp.org/PreBuilt/NSI_Role_Appendices.pdf; Copyright Ross Products Division of Abbott Laboratories; with permission.

Appendix 2: Instrumental activities of daily living (IADL) scale

Self-rated version extracted from the multilevel assessment instrument (MAI)

1. Can you use the telephone:
   without help,   3
   with some help, or   2
   are you completely unable to use the telephone?   1

2. Can you get to places out of walking distance:
   without help,   3
   with some help, or   2
   are you completely unable to travel unless special arrangement are made?   1

3. Can you go shopping for groceries:
   without help,   3
   with some help, or   2
   are you completely unable to do any shopping?   1

4. Can you prepare your own meals:
   without help,   3
   with some help, or   2
   are you completely unable to prepare any meals?   1

5. Can you do your own housework:
   without help,   3
   with some help, or   2
   are you completely unable to do any housework?   1

6. Can you do your own handyman work:
   without help,   3
   with some help, or   2
   are you completely unable to do any handyman work?   1

(continued on next page)

Appendix 2 (*continued*)

7. Can you do your own laundry:
   - without help,   3
   - with some help, or   2
   - are you completely unable to do any laundry at all?   1
8a. Do you take medicines or use any medications?
   - (If yes, answer Question 8b) Yes   1
   - (If no, answer Question 8c) No   2
8b. Do you take your own medicine
   - without help (in the right time),   3
   - with some help (take medicine if someone prepares it for   2
     you and/or reminds you to take it), or
   - (are you/would you be) completely unable to take your own medicine?   1
8c. If you had to take medicine, can you do it
   - without help (in the right doses at the right time),   3
   - with some help (take medicine if someone prepares it for you   2
     and/or reminds you to take it), or
   - (are you/would you be) completely unable to take your own medicine?   1
9. Can you manage your own money:
   - without help,   3
   - with some help, or   2
   - are you completely unable to handle money?   1

Modified from Lawton MP, Brody EM. Assessment of older people: self-maintaining and instrumental activities of daily living. Gerontologist 1969;9: 179–86; with permission.

Appendix 3a: Clock drawing task

The clock drawing task (CDT) is one of several commonly used screening tests for cognitive impairment. Inability to complete the task does not establish a diagnosis of dementia, but indicates that further testing is needed. Clock drawing is a complex tast that measures constructional skills and reflects how a person perceives time.

The CDT is administered by asking the patient to complete a freehand drawing of the face of a clock that shows the numbers and the hands with the hands indicating a time of 10 minutes to 11. The 0 to 4 scoring method is shown below:

Draws closed circle:	1 point
Numbers in correct position:	1 point
All 12 numbers:	1 point
Hands in correct position:	1 point

Distorted contour or extraneous markings are rarely produced by patients who are cognitively intact. Conversely, it is unlikely that a perfectly drawn clock will be produced by a cognitively impaired person.

Modified from Tuolcko H, Hadjistavropoulos T, Miller JA, et al. The clock test: a sensitive measure to differentiate normal elderly from those with Alzheimer disease. J Am Geriatr Soc 1992;40:1095–9; with permission.

Appendix 3b: Functional activities questionnaire

The FAQ is an informant-based measure of functional abilities. Informants provide performance ratings of the target person on 10 complex, higher-order activities.

Individual items of the functional activities questionnaire

1. Writing checks, paying bills, balancing a checkbook
2. Assembling tax records, business affairs, or papers
3. Shopping alone for clothes, household necessities, or groceries
4. Playing a game of skill, working on a hobby
5. Heating water, making a cup of coffee, turning off the stove
6. Preparing a balanced meal
7. Keeping track of current events
8. Paying attention to, understanding, discussing a TV show, book, or magazine
9. Remembering appointments, family occasions, holidays, medications
10. Traveling out of the neighborhood, driving, arranging to take buses

The levels of performance assigned range from dependence to independence, and are rated as follows:

Dependent = 3
Requires assistance = 2
Has difficulty but does by self = 1
Normal = 0

Two other response options can also be scored:

Never did (the activity), but could do now = 0
Never did and would have difficulty now = 1

A total score for the FAQ is computed by simply summing the scores across the 10 items. Scores range from 0 to 30; the higher the score, the poorer the function, ie, the greater the impairment. A cutpoint of 9 (dependent in 3 or more activities) is recommended.

Modified from Pfeffer RI, Kurosaki TT, Harrah CH, et al. Measurement of functional adults in the community. J Gerontol 1982;37:323–9; with permission.

Appendix 3c: Mini-mental state examination (MMSE)

Add points for each correct response.

		Score	Points
Orientation			
1. What is the:	Year?	—	2
	Season?	—	1
	Date?	—	1
	Day		
	Month?	—	1
2. Where are we?	State?	—	1
	County?	—	1
	Town or city?	—	1
	Hospital?	—	1
	Floor?	—	1
Registration			
3. Name three objects, taking one second to say each. Then ask the patient to repeat all three after you have said them. Give one point for each correct answer. Repeat the answers until patient learns all three.		—	3
Attention and calculation			
4. Serial sevens. Give one point for each correct answer. Stop after five answers. Alternate: spell WORLD backwards.		—	3
Recall			
5. Ask for names of three objects learned in question 3. Give one point for each correct answer.		—	3
Language			
6. Point to a pencil and a watch. Have the patient name them as you point.		—	2
7. Have the patient repeat "No ifs, ands, or buts."		—	1
8. Have the patient follow a three-stage command: "Take a paper in your right hand. Fold the paper in half. Put the paper on the floor."		—	3
9. Have the patient read and obey the following: "CLOSE YOUR EYES" (Write it in large letters.)		—	1
10. Have the patient write a sentence of his or her choice. (The sentence should contain a subject and an object and should make sense. Ignore spelling errors when scoring.)		—	1
11. Have the patient copy the design. (Give one point if all sides and angles are preserved and if the intersecting sides form a quandrangle.)		—	1

—	1
—	Total 30

In validation studies using a cut-off score of 23 or below, the MMSE has a sensitivity of 87%, a specificity of 82%, a false positive ratio of 39.4%, and a false negative ratio of 4.7%. These ratios refer to the MMSE's capacity to accurately distinguish patients with clinically diagnosed dementia or delirium from patients without these syndromes.

Modified from Folstein MF, Folstein S, McHugh PR. "Mini-mental state." A practical method for grading the cognitive state of patients for the clinician. J Psychiatr Res 1975;12:189–98; with permission.

Appendix 3d: DSM-IV criteria for dementia

Diagnostic criteria for dementia

A. The development of multiple cognitive deficits manifested by both

    (1) memory impairment (impaired ability to learn new information or to recall previously learned information)

    (2) one (or more) of the following cognitive disturbances:

        (a) aphasia (language disturbance)

        (b) apraxia (impaired ability to carry out motor activities despite intact motor function)

        (c) agnosia (failure to recognize or identify objects despite intact sensory function)

        (d) disturbance in executive functioning (ie, planning, organizing, sequencing, abstracting)

B. The cognitive deficits in criteria A1 and A2 each cause significant impairment in social or occupational functioning and represent a significant decline from a previous level of functioning.

C. The deficits do not occur exclusively during the course of a delirium.

D. The disturbance is not better accounted for by another axis 1 disorder (eg, major depressive disorder, schizophrenia).

Diagnostic criteria for dementia of the Alzheimer's type

A. The course is characterized by gradual onset and continuing cognitive decline.

B. The cognitive deficits in criteria A1 and A2 are not due to any of the following:

    (1) other central nervous system conditions that cause progressive deficits in memory and cognition (eg, cerebrovascular disease, Parkinson's disease, Huntington' disease, subdural hematoma, normal-pressure hydrocephalus, brain tumor)

    (2) systemic conditions that are known to cause dementia (eg, hypothyroidism, vitamin B_{12} or folic acid deficiency, niacin deficiency, hypercalcemia, neurosyphilis, HIV infection)

    (3) substance-induced conditions

Diagnostic criteria for vascular dementia

A. Focal neurological signs and symptoms (eg, exaggeration of deep tendon reflexes, extensor plantar response, pseudobulbar palsy, gait abnormalities, weakness of an extremity) or laboratory evidence indicative of cerebrovascular disease (eg, multiple infarctions involving cortex and underlying white matter) that are judged to be etiologically related to the disturbance.

B. The deficits do not occur exclusively during the course of a delirium.

Modified from American Psychiatric Association. Diagnostic and statistical manual of mental disorders (DSM-IV). 4th edition. Washington (DC): The American Psychiatric Association; 1994; with permission.

Appendix 3e: DSM-IV criteria for delirium

Diagnostic criteria for 293.0 delirium due to... [indicate the general medical condition]

A. Disturbance of consciousness (ie, reduced clarity of awareness of the environment) with reduced ability to focus, sustain, or shift attention.
B. A change in cognition (eg, memory deficit, disorientation, language disturbance) or the development of perceptual disturbance that is not better accounted for by a preexisting, established, or evolving dementia.
C. The disturbance develops over a short period of time (usually hours to days) and tends to fluctuate during the course of the day.
D. There is evidence from the history, physical examination, or laboratory findings that the disturbance is caused by the direct physiological consequences of a general medical condition.

Coding note: If delirium is superimposed on a pre-existing dementia of the Alzheimer's type or vascular dementia, indicate the delirium by coding the appropriate subtype of the dementia (eg, 290.3 dementia of the Alzheimer's type, with late onset, with delirium).

Coding note: Include the name of the general medical condition on axis I (eg, 293.0 delirium due to hepatic encephalopathy); also code the general medical condition on axis III.

Modified from American Psychiatric Association. Diagnostic and statistical manual of mental disorders (DSM-IV). 4th edition. Washington (DC): The American Psychiatric Association; 1994; with permission.

Appendix 4a: Get up and go test

- Sitting balance
- Arising from a chair
- Immediate standing balance
- Gait
- Turning balance
- Sitting into a chair

Standing

Does the person stand in a single slow motion? Does the person push up with their hands to get out of the chair? Are armrests helpful in getting out of the chair? Does the person need to move forward in the chair first? Does the person need to rock back and forth prior to standing up? Or, can the person stand with both hands crossed across his/her chest?

Is the person steady with standing or does it take a moment to gain balance? Does the person complain of dizziness or lightheadedness when they initially stand?

Walking

Does the person walk across the room without swaying or tottering? Is there a limp? Does the person hang on to furniture or other objects as they walk? Does the person require a cane or walker? Does the person lift their feet or shuffle?

Turning

Does the person remain steady with turning? Or, does the person totter? How many steps does it take to turn a corner?

Sitting

Does the person sit slowly and steadily? Or, does the person "plop" into a chair? Does the person land in the center of the chair or fall to one side?

Safety

Persons with cognitive impairment and physical impairments may require supervision to assure safety.

Modified from Tinetti ME, Ginter SF. Identifying mobility dysfuncions in elderly patients. Standard neuromuscular examination or direct assessment. JAMA 1988;259:1190–3, with permission; and Tinetti ME. Performance-oriented assessment of mobility problems in elderly patients. J Am Geriatr Soc 1986;34:119–26.

Appendix 4b: Performance-oriented mobility screen

Instructions: Ask the person to perform the following maneuvers. For each, indicate whether the person's performance is normal or abnormal.

Ask person to:	Observe:	Response:
1. Sit down in chair. Select a chair with armrests that is approximately 16–17 inches in seat height.	Able to sit down in one smooth, controlled movement without using armrests.	Normal
	Sitting is not a smooth movement; falls into chair or needs armrests to guide self into chair.	Abnormal
2. Rise up from chair.	Able to get up in one smooth, controlled movement without armrests.	Normal
	Uses armrests and/or moves forward in chair to proper self up; requires several attempts to get up.	Abnormal
3. Stand after rising from chair for approximately 30 seconds in place.	Steady; able to stand without support.	Normal
	Unsteady; loses balance	Abnormal
4. Stand with eyes closed for approximately 15 seconds in place.	Steady; able to stand without support.	Normal
	Unsteady; loses balance.	Abnormal
5. Stand with feet together, push lightly on sternum 2 to 3 times.	Steady; maintains balance.	Normal
	Unsteady; loses balance.	Abnormal
6. Reach up into tiptoes as if attempting to reach an object	Steady; maintains balance.	Normal
	Unsteady; loses balance.	Abnormal
7. Bend down as if attempting to obtain object from floor.	Steady, without loss of balance	Normal
	Unsteady; loses balance.	Abnormal

(continued on next page)

Appendix 4b (*continued*)

Instructions: If the person uses a walking aid such as a cane or walker, the following walking maneuvers are tested separately with and without the aid. Indicate type of aid used.

8. Walk in a straight line, in your "usual" pace (a distance approximately 15 feet); then walk back.	Gait is continuous without hesitation; walks in a straight line and both feet clear the floor.	Normal (with aid)
	Gait is noncontinuous with hesitation; deviates from straight path; feet scrape or shuffle on floor.	Abnormal (with aid)
		Abnormal (without aid)
9. Walk a distance of 5 feet and turn around.	Does not stagger; steps are smooth, continuous.	Normal (with aid)
		Normal (without aid)
	Staggers; steps are unsteady, discontinuous.	Abnormal (with aid)
		Abnormal (without aid)
10. Lie down on floor and get up.	Able to rise, without loss of balance.	Normal
	Unable to rise, or loses balance in the process.	Abnormal

Modified from Katz A, Ford AB, Moskowitz RW. Studies of illness in the aged. The index of ADL: a standardized measure of biological and psychosocial function. JAMA 1963;185:914–9; with permission.

Appendix 5a: Geriatric depression scale (short form)

Choose the best answer for how you felt over the past week.

1. Are you basically satisfied with your life?	yes/no
2. Have you dropped many of your activities and interests?	yes/no
3. Do you feel that your life is empty?	yes/no
4. Do you often get bored?	yes/no
5. Are you in good spirits most of the time?	yes/no
6. Are you afraid that something bad is going to happen to you?	yes/no
7. Do you feel happy most of the time?	yes/no
8. Do you often feel helpless?	yes/no
9. Do you prefer to stay at home, rather than going out and doing new things?	yes/no
10. Do you feel you have more problems with memory than most?	yes/no
11. Do you think it is wonderful to be alive now?	yes/no
12. Do you feel pretty worthless the way you are now?	yes/no
13. Do you feel full of energy?	yes/no
14. Do you feel that your situation is hopeless?	yes/no
15. Do you think that most people are better off than you are?	yes/no

This is the scoring for the scale. One point for each of these answers. Cut-off: normal (0–5); above 5 suggests depression.

1. no	6. yes	11. no
2. yes	7. no	12. yes
3. yes	8. yes	13. no
4. yes	9. yes	14. yes
5. no	10. yes	15. yes

Modified from Sheikh JI, Yesavage JA. Geriatric depression scale: recent evidence and development of a shorter version. Clin Gerontol 1986;5:165–72; with permission; and Yesavage JA, Brink TL, Rose TL, et al. Development and validation of a geriatric depression rating scale: a preliminary report. J Psych Res 1983;17:27.

Appendix 5b: DSM-IV criteria for major depression

1. Five (or more) of the following symptoms have been present during the same 2-week period and represent a change from previous functioning: at least one of the symptoms is either (1) depressed mood or (2) loss of interest or pleasure. (Note: Do not include symptoms that are clearly due to a general medical condition, or mood-incongruent delusions or hallucinations.)

    a. Depressed mood most of the day, nearly every day, as indicated by either subjective report (eg, feels sad or empty) or observation made by others (eg, appears tearful). Note: in children and adolescents, can be irritable mood.

    b. Markedly diminished interest or pleasure in all, or almost all, activities most of the day, nearly every day (as indicated by either subjective account or observation made by others).

    c. Significant weight loss while not dieting or weight gain (eg, a change of more than 5% of body weight in a month), or decrease or increase in appetite nearly every day. Note: In children, consider failure to make expected weight gains.

    d. Insomnia or hypersomnia nearly every day.

    e. Psychomotor agitation or retardation nearly every day (observable by others, not merely subjective feelings of restlessness or being slowed down).

    f. Fatigue or loss of energy nearly every day.

    g. Feelings of worthlessness or excessive or inappropriate guilt (which may be delusional) nearly every day (not merely self-reproach or guilt about being sick).

    h. Diminished ability to think or concentrate, or indecisiveness, nearly every day (either by subjective account or as observed by others).

    i. Recurrent thoughts of death (not just fear of dying), recurrent suicidal ideation without a specific plan, or a suicide attempt or a specific plan for committing suicide.

2. The symptoms do not meet criteria for a mixed episode.
3. The symptoms cause clinically significant distress or impairment in social, occupational, or other important areas of functioning.
4. The symptoms are not due to the direct physiological effects of a substance (eg, a drug of abuse, a medication) or a general medical condition (eg, hypothyroidism).

5. The symptoms are not better accounted for by bereavement; ie, after the loss of a loved one, the symptoms persist for longer than two months or are characterized by marked functional impairment, morbid preoccupation with worthlessness, suicidal ideation, psychotic symptoms, or psychomotor retardation.

Modified from American Psychiatric Association. Diagnostic and statistical manual of mental disorders (DSM-IV). 4th edition. Washington (DC): The American Psychiatric Association; 1994; with permission.

Appendix 5c: Cornell scale for depression in dementia

NAME_____AGE_____SEX_____DATE_____

WING_____ROOM_____PHYSICIAN_____ASSESSOR_____

Ratings should be based on symptoms and signs occurring during the week before interview. No score should be given if symptoms result from physical disability or illness.

Scoring System

a = Unable to evaluate   0 = Absent   1 = Mild to intermittent   2 = Severe

a	0	1	2	A. MOOD-RELATED SIGNS

A. MOOD-RELATED SIGNS
1. Anxiety: anxious expression, rumination, worrying
2. Sadness: sad expression, sad voice, tearfulness
3. Lack of reaction to present events
4. Irritability: annoyed, short tempered

a	0	1	2

B. BEHAVIORAL DISTURBANCE
5. Agitation: restlessness, hand wringing, hair pulling
6. Retardation: slow movements, slow speech, slow reactions
7. Multiple physical complaints (score 0 if gastrointestinal symptoms only)
8. Loss of interest: less involved in usual activities (score only if change occurred acutely, ie, in less than one month)

a	0	1	2

C. PHYSICAL SIGNS
9. Appetile loss: eating less than usual
10. Weight loss (score 2 if greater than 5 pounds in one month)
11. Lack of energy: faligues easily, unable to sustain activities

a	0	1	2

D. CYCLIC FUNCTIONS
12. Diurnal variation of mood: symptoms worse in the morning
13. Difficulty falling asleep: later than usual for this individual
14. Multiple awakening during sleep
15. Early morning awakening: earlier than usual for this individual

a	0	1	2

E. IDEATIONAL DISTURBANCE
16. Suicidal: feels life is not worth living
17. Poor self-esteem: self-blame, self-depreciation, feelings of failure
18. Pessimism: anticipation of the worst
19. Mood congruent delusions: delusions of poverty, illness, or loss

SCORE_____ Score greater than 12 = probable depression

Notes/current/medications:_____

_____

_____

Modified from Alexopoulos GS, Abrams RC, Young RC, et al. Cornell scale for depression in dementia. Biol Psychiatry 1988;23:271–84.

Appendix 6a: Michigan alcoholism screening test—geriatric version (MAST-G)

1. After drinking, have you ever noticed an increase in your heart or beating in your chest?
2. When talking with others, do you ever underestimate how much you actually drink?
3. Does alcohol make you sleepy so that you often fall asleep in your chair?
4. After a few drinks, have you sometimes not eaten or been able to skip a meal because you don't feel hungry?
5. Does having a few drinks help decrease your shakiness or tremors?
6. Does alcohol sometimes make it hard for you to remember parts of the day or night?
7. Do you have rules for yourself that you won't drink before a certain time of the day?
8. Have you lost interest in hobbies or activities you used to enjoy?
9. When you wake up in the morning, do you ever have trouble remembering part of the night before?
10. Does having a drink help you to sleep?
11. Do you hide your alcohol bottles from your family members?
12. After a social gathering, have you ever felt embarrassed because you drank too much?
13. Have you ever been concerned that drinking might be harmful to your health?
14. Do you like to end an evening with a nightcap?
15. Did you find your drinking increased after someone close to you died?
16. In general, would you prefer to have a few drinks at home rather than go out to social events?
17. Are you drinking more now than in the past?
18. Do you usually take a drink to relax or calm your nerves?
19. Do you drink to take your mind off your problems?
20. Have you ever increased your drinking after experiencing a loss in your life?
21. Do you sometimes drive when you have had too much to drink?
22. Has a doctor or nurse ever said they were worried or concerned about your drinking?
23. Have you ever made rules to manage your drinking?
24. When you feel lonely, does having a drink help?

Scoring: 5 or more "yes" responses is indicative of an alcohol problem.

Modified from Blow FC, Cook CA, Booth BM, et al. Alcohol, MAST-G. Clin Exp Res 1992;116:372.

Appendix 6b: The CAGE questionnaire

1. Have you ever felt you could Cut down on your drinking?
2. Have people Annoyed you by criticizing your drinking?
3. Have you felt bad or Guilty about your drinking?
4. Have you ever had a drink first thing in the morning to steady your nerves or get rid of a hangover? (Eyeopener)

Modified from Ewing J. Detecting alcoholism: the CAGE questionnaire. JAMA 1989;252:510.

Appendix 7a: Zarit burden interview

Instruction given to caregiver: *The following is a list of statements that reflect how persons sometimes feel when taking care of another person. After each statement, indicate how often you feel that way never, rarely, sometimes, quite frequently, or nearly always. There are no right or wrong answers.*

	Never	Rarely	Sometimes	Quite Frequently	Nearly Always
	0	1	2	3	4
1. Do you feel that your relative asks for more help than he/she needs?	☐	☐	☐	☐	☐
2. Do you feel that because of the time you spend with your relative that you don't have enough time for yourself?	☐	☐	☐	☐	☐
3. Do you feel stressed between caring for your relative and trying to meet other responsibilities for your family or work?	☐	☐	☐	☐	☐
4. Do you feel embarrassed over your relative's behavior?	☐	☐	☐	☐	☐
5. Do you feel angry when you are around your relative?	☐	☐	☐	☐	☐
6. Do you feel that your relative currently affects yours relationship with other family members or friends in a negative way?	☐	☐	☐	☐	☐
7. Are you afraid what the future holds for your relative?	☐	☐	☐	☐	☐
8. Do you feel your relative is dependent on you?	☐	☐	☐	☐	☐
9. Do you feel strained when you are around your relative?	☐	☐	☐	☐	☐
10. Do you feel your health has suffered because of your involvement with your relative?	☐	☐	☐	☐	☐
11. Do you feel that you don't have as much privacy as you would like because of your relative?	☐	☐	☐	☐	☐
12. Do you feel that your social life has suffered because you are caring for your relative?	☐	☐	☐	☐	☐
13. Do you feel uncomfortable about having friends over because of your relative?	☐	☐	☐	☐	☐
14. Do you feel that your relative seems to expect you to take care of him/her as if you were the only one he/she could depend on?	☐	☐	☐	☐	☐
15. Do you feel that you don't have enough money to care for your relative in addition to the rest of your expenses?	☐	☐	☐	☐	☐

16. Do you feel that you will be unable to   ☐   ☐   ☐   ☐   ☐
    take care of your relative much longer?
17. Do you feel you have lost   ☐   ☐   ☐   ☐   ☐
    control of your life since your
    relative's illness?
18. Do you wish you could leave the care of   ☐   ☐   ☐   ☐   ☐
    your relative to someone else?
19. Do you feel uncertain about what to   ☐   ☐   ☐   ☐   ☐
    do about your relative?
20. Do you feel you should be doing more   ☐   ☐   ☐   ☐   ☐
    for your relative?
21. Do you feel you could do a better   ☐   ☐   ☐   ☐   ☐
    job in caring for your relative?
22. Overall, how often do you feel   ☐   ☐   ☐   ☐   ☐
    burdened in caring for your relative?
              Total Score In Each Column   —   —   —   —   —

                    GRAND TOTAL   ——

Comments:_____
_____
_____
_____
_____
_____

_____

Modified from Zarit SH, Reever K, Bach-Peterson J. Relatives of the impaired elderly:
correlates of burden. Gerontologist 1980;20:649–55.

Appendix 7b: The caregiver strain questionnaire

I am going to read a list of things which other people have found to be difficult in helping out after somebody comes home from the hospital. Would you tell me whether any of these apply to you?
(GIVE EXAMPLES)

	Yes = 1	No = 0
Sleep is disturbed (eg, because ____ is in and out of bed or wanders around at night)	—	—
It is inconvenient (eg, because helping takes so much time or it's a long drive over to help)	—	—
It is a physical strain (eg, because of lifting in and out of a chair; effort or concentration is required)	—	—
It is confining (eg, helping restricts free time or cannot go visiting)	—	—
There have been family adjustments (eg, because helping has disrupted routine; there has been no privacy)	—	—
There have been changes in personal plans (eg, had to turn down a job; could not go on vacation)	—	—
There have been other demands on my time (eg, from other family members)	—	—
There have been emotional adjustments (eg, because of severe arguments)	—	—
Some behavior is upsetting (eg, because of incontinence; ___ has trouble remembering things; or ___ accuses people of taking things)	—	—
It is upsetting to find ___ has changed so much from his/her former self (eg, he/she is a different person than he/she used to be)	—	—
There have been work adjustments (eg, because of having to take time off)	—	—
It is a financial strain	—	—
Feeling completely overwhelmed (eg, because of worry about ___; concerns about how you will manage)	—	—
Total score (count yes responses)	—	—

Modified from Robinson B. Validation of a caregiver strain index. J Gerontol 1983;38:344–8; with permission.

Appendix 8: Environment—home safety checklist

Food supply/preparation

Adequate/appropriate supply of food	Y	N
Kitchen adequate for food preparation	Y	N
Cooking utensils adequate/appropriate	Y	N

Medication(s)

Does patient have prescription medications	Y	N
Medications marked clearly	Y	N
Medications stored properly	Y	N
Prescriptions current	Y	N
Medication given by:	Patient Caregiver	
If patient takes own medication, able to verbalize or demonstrate appropriate use:	Y	N
Number of prescription medications patient is currently taking ___ (write in)		

Neighborhood

Location (circle one)	Urban	Suburban	Rural
High crime/unsafe	Y	N	

Physical hazards

Sturdy handrails/banisters by all steps/stairs	Y N N/A (no stairs)
Adequate lighting in all hallways and stairs	Y N
Light switch at both top and bottom of stairs	Y N N/A (no stairs)
Pathways, hallways, stairways clear of clutter and loose objects	Y N
Flashlight, lightswitch, or lamp beside bed or nightlight in bathroom/hallway	Y N
Electric cords close to walls, out of pathways	Y N
Lightswitch by doorway of each room	Y N
Rugs secure around all edges; rugs smooth and flat with no wrinkles	Y N
Phone easily accessible	Y N N/A (no phone)
List of emergency numbers by phone/clearly visible	Y N N/A (no phone)
Gas pipes and major appliances in good repair	Y N
Home adequately heated, ventilated, insulated	Y N
Non-skid surface on floor of shower/tub	Y N
Adequate hand-holds for getting in and out of tub	Y N N/A (doesn't use tub)
Adequate hand-holds for sitting and rising from toilet	Y N
Smoke detector in home	Y N

ELSEVIER
SAUNDERS

Prim Care Clin Office Pract
32 (2005) 855–864

PRIMARY CARE:
CLINICS IN
OFFICE PRACTICE

Index

Note: Page numbers of article titles are in **boldface** type.

Changing Your Address?

Make sure your subscription changes too! When you notify us of your new address, you can help make our job easier by including an exact copy of your Clinics label number with your old address (see illustration below.) This number identifies you to our computer system and will speed the processing of your address change. Please be sure this label number accompanies your old address and your corrected address—you can send an old Clinics label with your number on it or just copy it exactly and send it to the address listed below.

We appreciate your help in our attempt to give you continuous coverage. Thank you.

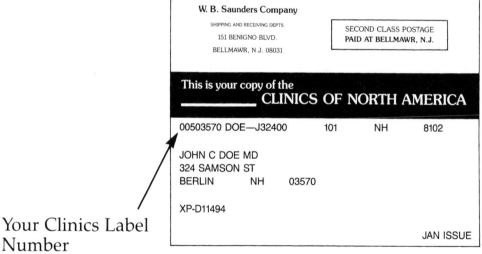

Your Clinics Label Number
Copy it exactly or send your label
along with your address to:
W.B. Saunders Company, Customer Service
Orlando, FL 32887-4800
Call Toll Free 1-800-654-2452

Please allow four to six weeks for delivery of new subscriptions and for processing address changes.